Traditional Mediterranean Di

Delicious and Wholesome Recipes to Live

TABLE OF CONTENTS

INTRODUCTION

There is an abundance of ways to follow the Mediterranean diet. The beauty of this way of eating is the liberty it provides when it comes to food choices. There are guidelines, but they are not as strict as some other diets. Let's list the main foods and drinks you will eat if you go Mediterranean:

Fruits and Vegetables

You can't imagine a Mediterranean meal without vegetables, and if you see someone from the Mediterranean snacking, it is probably on fruit. Fruits and vegetables might be the main reason this diet works so well. Not only are they rich in fiber and therefor satiating and gut-friendly, they also carry a plethora of vitamins and minerals.

You should stock up on leafy greens that will be the base for most of your salads. There is lettuce, spinach, arugula, and watercress, and you can also try corn salad and Chinese cabbage.

For fruit and other vegetables, you can't go wrong, as long as it is fresh and has no added sugar. There is no fruit that is less Mediterranean than another. However, people in the Mediterranean usually eat seasonal fruit and vegetables, so you might want to consider that if you are someone who craves tomato in December and ends up eating something that vaguely resembles a tomato at a huge price. Not only are seasonal fruits and vegetables more budget friendly, they are usually healthier, tastier and easier to find.

Red Meat and Red Wine

People from the Mediterranean have never eaten much pork or beef. This might be because they did not have much cattle, or because bovines were more useful working in the field than as food (the terrain was pretty unforgiving), but regardless of the reason, people ate less meat from pigs, cows and goats.

For this reason, people from the Mediterranean have a much lower risk of developing diabetes or cardiovascular diseases. Red meat contains saturated fats and is high in calories, especially when compared to seafood, fish and legumes.

Before you ditch the red meat altogether, it is not all bad. Red meat is higher in creatine than other meats, and it contains minerals that are otherwise difficult to consume in large quantities. Just keep your consumption moderate.

Red wine is pretty much the same deal. It is not inherently bad, but people tend to misuse it too often for doctors to recommend it in good conscience. It is understandable why people think that wine is an irreplaceable part of the Mediterranean diet. After all, almost every movie or picture showcasing this part of the world has somebody reaching for a bottle of good old red.

Like with most things, the takeaway with red wine is not that alcohol is bad in and of itself, but rather that you should limit the amount you consume if you want to reap the benefits without the adverse effects. The general guideline is to keep your alcohol consumption under 14 units per week.

Eggs and Dairy

Eggs and dairy are not forbidden in the Mediterranean diet, but they are to be eaten in moderation. I am not saying eggs and dairy are bad for you, but people on the Mediterranean diet curb them because their fat requirements are already met through olive oil, oily fish, seafood, avocado, seeds and nuts. However, you can still eat them from time to time. Eggs are versatile, affordable, and a complete protein.

Milk is another thing we try to consume in smaller quantities when following this diet, but there are some milk products that are quite common in the Mediterranean diet, such as Greek yoghurt, kefir and fresh cheese.

Fish and Seafood

Fish and seafood are an amazing source of complete protein that comes cheap calorie wise. They are also a rich source of healthy fatty acids, most notably omega-3s. Depending on where you live, some fish may be easier or more difficult to find, but remember to include both white fish (richer in protein) and red fish (richer in healthy fats) in your diet.

Olive Oil, Herbs and Spices

Olive oil can fit into the previous category as it is another source of healthy fats, but it deserves a place of its own, due to its popularity and prevalence in this diet. Indeed, it is difficult to imagine a single Mediterranean dish that doesn't include olive oil.

Oleic acid, the largest part (3/4) of olive oil has many proven health benefits, most famously, reducing inflammation and decreasing the risk of cancer (it has beneficial effects on genes linked to cancer, and a high number of antioxidants). Additionally, olive oil can promote brain health and improve cognitive function, and it has antibacterial properties.

Herbs and spices are in this category because they go hand in hand with olive oil. Also, they are part of the reason the Mediterranean diet is so healthy. One thing we don't lack in this day and age is sodium. Yes, we need it, but not nearly as much as we tend to consume. Replacing salt with spices and herbs can make a big difference, not only from curbing the amount of sodium we consume, but also because of the health benefits of herbs and spices such as basil, parsley, sage, saffron, rosemary, thyme and oregano.

Nuts and Seeds

Nuts and seeds are a staple food in many diets, due to their high protein and healthy fat content. Almonds, walnuts, cashews, sunflower seeds, pumpkin seeds, chia seeds and Brazil nuts all make excellent allies in the fight for brain health and longevity.

Not only are they rich in antioxidants and fiber, they are also rich in vitamins and minerals that most of us lack. For a long time, nuts and seeds had a bad rep due to the misconception that fats make you fat. Now that we know caloric surplus is what makes us gain weight, healthy fats are back in the game. It's always a bad idea to exclude an entire food group from your diet, and fats have been banished for far too long. Fats are important for our general health, but especially our heart, brain and eyesight.

Grains and Legumes

Combining grains and legumes will in most cases give us a complete protein (containing all or most of the nine essential amino acids). We all need protein to gain muscle and lose weight the right way.

Most people rely on meat, eggs and dairy for their main protein sources. However, people from the Mediterranean found that it's best to limit their meat intake and opt for grains and legumes instead.

Nowadays you can choose from a myriad of grains, but some of the most popular are:

Oats – a cheap and healthy option for a healthy gut, rich in protein and antioxidants. (Whenever you can, make your own oatmeal, instead of eating the pre-made ones, as they tend to be much higher in sugar). Oats can taste great with both sweet and savory foods added.

Quinoa – not only is quinoa rich in protein, it is also among the most complete plant proteins. It can be expensive in some parts of the world, so feel free to trade it for something else if you are on a tight budget.

Buckwheat – if you suffer from a gluten intolerance or sensitivity, buckwheat is the way to go. Not only is it gluten free, its protein profile is similar to that of quinoa, making it a powerful tool for building muscle. Buckwheat flour is a great replacement for wheat flour, so be sure to give buckwheat crepes a try.

Millet – rich in vitamins and higher in healthy fats than other grains, millet is also a clear choice for anybody with respiratory issues, such as asthma, as it doesn't contain the common allergens found in other grains. One interesting way to include millet in your diet is in a soup. Trust me, it's fantastic.

Barley – as it contains beta-glucan, a simple carb that our body can't digest, barley has long been known to keep insulin from spiking after big meals. Barley tea is popular in Italy, but you can use it in your cooking as well.

Combining grains with legumes can provide you with a complete protein, but it can also be an interesting cooking experience. You can't go wrong with choosing legumes you like, but it's important to change them up a bit once in a while, so you don't end up always eating the same thing. There are so many choices:

Peas – rich in protein and fiber, peas are as healthy as they are cheap, versatile and tasty. They also promote gut health, especially in elderly people. When buying fresh peas, look for the ones that are colored light green; they are younger and often tastier. Dark green old ones can be chewy and bitter.

Beans – they are all highly satiating, rich in protein and low in calories. Most of them are cheap, too. So, don't scratch your head over choosing the best bean among navy, pinto, black, or plain old kidney beans. Find that ones that are the most affordable, or the ones that you like most. Eventually you can try them all, see what you like, and mix them up every now and then.

Chickpeas – there is not a big difference between chickpeas and other legumes when it comes to health benefits. They, too, can help lower cholesterol, promote weight loss, and support gut health and insulin sensitivity.

What makes chickpeas special is their texture. They taste quite different from other legumes, and as such they make a great choice for salads, or when you get tired of eating the same thing over and over again.

Poultry

Poultry, such as chicken and turkey, is not a huge part of the Mediterranean diet. This doesn't mean that you can't have chicken at all;

you can eat more of it than red meat. It's lower in calories and unhealthy fats, and is a good source of protein with a high biological value.

Given that the meat industry is not the most responsible (especially in developing countries where laws are less rigid and regulations are not followed as closely), I always encourage people to find cage-free, organic, grass-fed chicken or turkey.

Lemon Juice Water

One of the simplest ways in which you can enrich your daily eating and exercise plan is to drink more water. The body often confuses when it is actually craving water rather than food. If you drink more water, then your stomach is going to feel fuller and you will be more hydrated, particularly in the summer months more than anything else.

The advantage of drinking water to other carbonated drinks and even fruit juices is that you are not giving your body more calories than are needed. You could add some squash to your water which can apparently help to rehydrate you quicker but generally it is better to stick to water. You can always add some ice and lemon for a fresher taste or even some lime. There are some associated health benefits to adding lemon or lime to your water which is a latest craze. The citrus fruits can give your body some Vitamin C and the potassium is another health benefit. This allows the body to be able to absorb vitamins and give your immune system a kick start in the morning in particular. It will help to absorb your breakfast.

BREAKFAST RECIPES

1. Mediterranean Frittata

Preparation Time: 8 minutes

Cooking Time: 6 minutes

Servings: 4

INGREDIENTS:

- 2 teaspoons of olive oil
- 3/4 cup of baby spinach, packed
- 2 green onions
- 4 egg whites, large
- 6 large eggs
- 1/3 cup of crumbled feta cheese, (1.3 ounces) along with sun-dried tomatoes and basil
- 2 teaspoons of salt-free Greek seasoning
- 1/4 teaspoon of salt

DIRECTIONS:

1. Take a boiler and preheat it. Take a ten-inch ovenproof skillet and pour the oil into it and keep the skillet on a medium flame.
2. While the oil gets heated, chop the spinach roughly and the onions. Put the eggs, egg whites, Greek seasoning, cheese, as well as salt in a large mixing bowl and mix it thoroughly using a whisker.

3. Add the chopped spinach and onions into the mixing bowl and stir it well.

4. Pour the mixture into the pan and cook it for 2 minutes or more until the edges of the mixture set well.

5. Lift the edges of the mixture gently and tilt the pan so that the uncooked portion can get underneath it. Cook for another two minutes so that the whole mixture gets cooked properly.

6. Broil for two to three minutes till the center gets set. Your Frittata is now ready. Serve it hot by cutting it into four wedges.

NUTRITION: Calories: 178 Protein: 16 g Fat: 12 g Carbs: 2.2 g

2. Honey-Caramelized Figs with Greek Yogurt

Preparation Time: 5 minutes

Cooking Time: 5 minutes

Servings: 4

INGREDIENTS:

- 4 fresh halved figs
- 2 tablespoons of melted butter, 30ml
- 2 tablespoons of brown sugar, 30ml
- 2 cups of Greek yogurt 500ml
- 1/4 cup of honey, 60ml

DIRECTIONS:

1. Take a non-stick skillet and preheat it over a medium flame. Put the butter on the pan and toss the figs into it and sprinkle in some brown sugar over it.

2. Put the figs on the pan and cut off the side of the figs. Cook the figs on a medium flame for 2-3 minutes until they turn a golden brown.

3. Turn over the figs and cook them for 2-3 minutes again. Remove the figs from the pan and let it cool down a little.

4. Take a plate and put a scoop of Greek yogurt on it. Put the cooked figs over the yogurts and drizzle the honey over it

NUTRITION: Calories: 350 Protein: 6 g Fat: 19 g Carbs: 40 g

3. Savory Quinoa Egg Muffins with Spinach

Preparation Time: 15 minutes

Cooking Time: 20 minutes

Servings: 2

INGREDIENTS:

- 1 cup of quinoa
- 2 cups of water/ vegetable broth)
- 4 ounces of spinach which is about one cup
- 1/2 chopped onion
- 2 whole eggs
- 1/4 cup of grated cheese
- 1/2 teaspoon of oregano or thyme
- 1/2 teaspoon of garlic powder

- 1/2 teaspoon of salt

DIRECTIONS:

1. Take a medium saucepan and put water in it. Add the quinoa in the water and bring the whole thing to a simmer.

2. Cover the pan and cook it for 10 minutes till the water gets absorbed by the quinoa. Remove the saucepan from the heat and let it cool down.

3. Take a nonstick pan and heat the onions till they turn soft and then add spinach. Cook all of them together till the spinach gets a little wilted and then remove it from the heat.

4. Preheat the oven to 176 C. Take a muffin pan and grease it lightly.

5. Take a large bowl and add the cooked quinoa along with the cooked onions, spinach, and add cheese, eggs, thyme or oregano, salt, garlic powder, pepper and mix them together.

6. Put a spoonful of the mixture into a muffin tin. Make sure it is ¼ of a cup. In the preheated pan, put it in the pan and bake it for around 20 minutes.

NUTRITION: Calories: 61 Protein: 4 g Fat: 3 g Carbs: 6 g

4. Avocado Tomato Gouda Socca Pizza

Preparation Time: 20 minutes

Cooking Time: 20 minutes

Servings: 2

INGREDIENTS:

- 1 and 1/4 cups of chickpea or garbanzo bean flour

- 1 and 1/4 cups of cold water
- 1/4 teaspoon of pepper and sea salt each
- 2 teaspoons of avocado or olive oil + 1 teaspoon extra for heating the pan
- 1 teaspoon of minced Garlic which will be around two cloves
- 1 teaspoon of Onion powder/other herb seasoning powder
- 10 to twelve-inch cast iron pan
- 1 sliced tomato
- 1/2 avocado
- 2 ounces of thinly sliced Gouda
- 1/4-1/3 cup of Tomato sauce
- 2 or 3 teaspoons of chopped green scallion/onion
- Sprouted greens for green
- Extra pepper/salt for sprinkling on top of the pizza
- Red pepper flakes

DIRECTIONS:

1. Mix the flour with two teaspoons of olive oil, herbs, water, and whisk it until a smooth mixture form. Keep it at room temperature for around 15-20 minutes to let the batter settle.

2. In the meantime, preheat the oven and place the pan inside the oven and let it get heated for around 10 minutes. When the pan gets preheated, chop up the vegetables into fine slices.

3. Remove the pan after ten minutes using oven mitts. Put one teaspoon of oil and swirl it all around to coat the pan.

4. Pour the batter into the pan and tilt the pan so that the batter spreads evenly throughout the pan. Turn down the over to 425f and place back the pan for 5-8 minutes.

5. Remove the pan from the oven and add the sliced avocado, tomato and on top of that, add the gouda slices and the onion slices.

6. Put the pizza back into the oven and wait till the cheese get melted or the sides of the bread gets crusty and brown.

7. Remove the pizza from the pan and add the microgreens on top, along with the toppings.

NUTRITION: Calories: 416 Protein: 15 g Fat: 10 g Carbs: 37 g

5. Sunny-Side Up Baked Eggs with Swiss Chard, Feta, and Basil

Preparation Time: 15 minutes

Cooking Time: 10 minutes

Servings: 4

INGREDIENTS:

- 4 bell peppers, any color
- 1 tablespoon extra-virgin olive oil
- 8 large eggs
- ¾ teaspoon kosher salt, divided
- ¼ teaspoon freshly ground black pepper, divided
- 1 avocado, peeled, pitted, and diced
- ¼ cup red onion, diced

- ¼ cup fresh basil, chopped
- Juice of ½ lime

DIRECTIONS:

1. Stem and seed the bell peppers. Cut 2 (2-inch-thick) rings from each pepper. Chop the remaining bell pepper into small dice and set aside.

2. Heat the olive oil in a large skillet over medium heat. Add 4 bell pepper rings, then crack 1 egg in the middle of each ring.

3. Season with ¼ teaspoon of the salt and 1/8 teaspoon of the black pepper. Cook until the egg whites are mostly set, but the yolks are still runny 2 to 3 minutes.

4. Gently flip and cook 1 additional minute for over easy. Move the egg–bell pepper rings to a platter or onto plates and repeats with the remaining 4 bell pepper rings.

5. In a medium bowl, combine the avocado, onion, basil, lime juice, reserved diced bell pepper, the remaining ¼ teaspoon kosher salt, and the remaining 1/8 teaspoon black pepper. Divide among the 4 plates.

NUTRITION: Calories: 270 Protein: 15 g Fat: 19 g Carbs: 12 g

6. Polenta with Sautéed Chard and Fried Eggs

Preparation Time: 5 minutes

Cooking Time: 20 minutes

Servings: 4

INGREDIENTS:

- 2½ cups water
- ½ teaspoon kosher salt
- ¾ cups whole-grain cornmeal
- ¼ teaspoon freshly ground black pepper
- 2 tablespoons grated Parmesan cheese
- 1 tablespoon extra-virgin olive oil
- 1 bunch (about 6 ounces) Swiss chard, leaves and stems chopped and separated
- 2 garlic cloves, sliced
- ¼ teaspoon kosher salt
- 1/8 teaspoon freshly ground black pepper
- Lemon juice (optional)
- 1 tablespoon extra-virgin olive oil
- 4 large eggs

DIRECTIONS:

1. For the polenta, bring the water and salt to a boil in a medium saucepan over high heat. Slowly add the cornmeal, whisking constantly.

2. Decrease the heat to low, cover, and cook for 10 to 15 minutes, stirring often to avoid lumps. Stir in the pepper and Parmesan and divide among 4 bowls.

3. For the chard, heat the oil in a large skillet over medium heat. Add the chard stems, garlic, salt, and pepper; sauté for 2 minutes. Add the chard leaves and cook until wilted, about 3 to 5 minutes.

4. Add a spritz of lemon juice (if desired), toss together, and divide evenly on top of the polenta.

5. For the eggs, heat the oil in the same large skillet over medium-high heat. Crack each egg into the skillet, taking care not to crowd the skillet and leaving space between the eggs.

6. Cook until the whites are set and golden around the edges, about 2 to 3 minutes. Serve sunny-side up or flip the eggs over carefully and cook 1 minute longer for over easy. Place one egg on top of the polenta and chard in each bowl.

NUTRITION: Calories: 310 Protein: 17 g Fat: 18 g Carbs: 21 g

7. Smoked Salmon Egg Scramble with Dill and Chives

Preparation Time: 5 minutes

Cooking Time: 5 minutes

Servings: 2

INGREDIENTS:

- 4 large eggs
- 1 tablespoon milk
- 1 tablespoon fresh chives, minced
- 1 tablespoon fresh dill, minced
- ¼ teaspoon kosher salt
- 1/8 teaspoon freshly ground black pepper
- 2 teaspoons extra-virgin olive oil
- 2 ounces smoked salmon, thinly sliced

DIRECTIONS:

1. In a large bowl, whisk together the eggs, milk, chives, dill, salt, and pepper. Heat the olive oil in a medium skillet or sauté pan over medium heat.

2. Add the egg mixture and cook for about 3 minutes, stirring occasionally. Add the salmon and cook until the eggs are set but moist about 1 minute.

NUTRITION: Calories: 325 Protein: 23 g Fat: 26 g Carbs: 1 g

8. Eggs with Zucchini Noodles

Preparation Time: 10 minutes

Cooking Time: 11 minutes

Servings: 2

INGREDIENTS:

- 2 tablespoons extra-virgin olive oil
- 3 zucchinis, cut with a spiralizer
- 4 eggs
- Salt and black pepper to the taste
- A pinch of red pepper flakes
- Cooking spray
- 1 tablespoon basil, chopped

DIRECTIONS:

1. In a bowl, combine the zucchini noodles with salt, pepper, and the olive oil, and toss well. Grease a baking sheet with cooking spray and divide the zucchini noodles into 4 nests on it.

2. Crack an egg on top of each nest, sprinkle salt, pepper, and the pepper flakes on top, and bake at 350 degrees F for 11 minutes. Divide the mix between plates, sprinkle the basil on top, and serve.

NUTRITION: Calories: 296 Protein: 15 g Fat: 24 g Carbs: 11 g

9. Banana Oats

Preparation Time: 10 minutes

Cooking Time: 0 minutes

Servings: 2

INGREDIENTS:

- 1 banana, peeled and sliced
- ¾ cup almond milk
- ½ cup cold-brewed coffee
- 2 dates, pitted
- 2 tablespoons cocoa powder
- 1 cup rolled oats
- 1 and ½ tablespoons chia seeds

DIRECTIONS:

1. In a blender, combine the banana with the milk and the rest of the ingredients, pulse, divide into bowls and serve for breakfast.

NUTRITION: Calories: 451 Protein: 9 g Fat: 25 g Carbs: 55 g

10. Slow-Cooked Peppers Frittata

Preparation Time: 10 minutes

Cooking Time: 3 hours

Servings: 6

INGREDIENTS:

- ½ cup almond milk
- 8 eggs, whisked
- Salt and black pepper to the taste
- 1 teaspoon oregano, dried
- 1 and ½ cups roasted peppers, chopped
- ½ cup red onion, chopped
- 4 cups baby arugula
- 1 cup goat cheese, crumbled
- Cooking spray

DIRECTIONS:

1. In a bowl, combine the eggs with salt, pepper, and the oregano and whisk. Grease your slow cooker with the cooking spray, arrange the peppers and the remaining ingredients inside and pour the egg mixture over them.
2. Put the lid on and cook on Low for 3 hours. Divide the frittata between plates and serve.

NUTRITION: Calories: 259 Protein: 16 g Fat: 20 g Carbs: 4.4 g

SALAD RECIPES

11. Spring Greek Salad

Preparation time: 15 minutes

Cooking time: 0 minutes

Servings: 4

INGREDIENTS:

- 1 head escarole, chopped
- 1 head curly chicory, chopped
- ¼ cup crumbled feta cheese
- ¼ cup pitted halved kalamata olives
- ¼ cup sliced seeded pepperoncini
- 3 tablespoons extra-virgin olive oil
- Juice of ½ lemon
- 2 garlic cloves, minced
- Pinch dried dill
- Salt
- Freshly ground black pepper

DIRECTIONS:

1. In a large bowl, toss together the escarole and chicory. Scatter the feta cheese, olives, and pepperoncini on top.

2. In a small bowl, whisk together the olive oil, lemon juice, and garlic. Season with the dill and salt and pepper to taste. Pour the dressing over the lettuce mixture and toss to combine.

NUTRITION: Calories: 173 Fat: 14g Protein: 5g Carbohydrates: 10g

12. Panzanella

Preparation time: 15 minutes

Cooking time: 10 minutes

Servings: 6

INGREDIENTS:

- ¼ cup extra-virgin olive oil, plus 3 tablespoons
- 6 stale hearty Italian bread slices, cut into cubes
- 6 tomatoes, cut into 1-inch pieces
- 1 cucumber, halved lengthwise and cut into half-moons
- 1 red bell pepper, seeded and finely chopped
- ½ onion, thinly sliced
- 2 tablespoons roughly chopped capers
- 2 tablespoons red wine vinegar
- 1 garlic clove, minced
- 1 teaspoon salt
- ¼ teaspoon freshly ground black pepper
- 1 teaspoon chopped fresh basil

DIRECTIONS:

1. In a large skillet, heat 3 tablespoons of olive oil over medium heat. Add the bread cubes and cook for about 10 minutes, until browned on all sides.

2. Transfer the bread cubes to a large bowl and add the tomatoes, cucumber, bell pepper, onion, and capers.

3. In a small bowl, whisk together the remaining ¼ cup of olive oil, the vinegar, garlic, salt, and pepper. Pour the dressing over the salad and toss to combine well.

4. Let the salad rest for 30 minutes. Sprinkle the basil on top and serve.

NUTRITION: Calories: 205 Fat: 17g Protein: 3g Carbohydrates: 13g

13. Tuscan Tuna Salad

Preparation time: 15 minutes

Cooking time: 0 minutes

Servings: 4

INGREDIENTS:

- ¼ cup extra-virgin olive oil
- Juice of ½ lemon
- ½ teaspoon Dijon mustard
- Salt
- Freshly ground black pepper
- 2 (5-ounce) cans tuna in olive oil, drained
- 1 (19-ounce) can cannellini beans, rinsed and drained
- 12 marinated mushrooms, rinsed and halved if large

- 12 grape or cherry tomatoes, halved
- 1 or 2 celery stalks, sliced
- 1 teaspoon capers (optional)

DIRECTIONS:

1. In a small bowl, whisk together the olive oil, lemon juice, and mustard, and season with salt and pepper.
2. In a large bowl, combine the tuna, beans, mushrooms, tomatoes, celery, and capers (if using). Add the dressing and toss well. Season with additional salt and pepper, if desired.

NUTRITION: Calories: 389 Fat: 20g Protein: 26g Carbohydrates: 29g

14. Mediterranean Chopped Salad

Preparation time: 15 minutes

Cooking time: 20 minutes

Servings: 4

INGREDIENTS:

- 1 cup whole grains, such as red or white quinoa, millet, or buckwheat
- 1 (15-ounce) can chickpeas, rinsed and drained
- 2 cups baby spinach
- 1 cucumber, finely chopped
- ½ red bell pepper, finely chopped
- ½ fennel bulb, trimmed and finely chopped
- 1 celery stalk, finely chopped
- 1 carrot, finely chopped

- 1 plum tomato, finely chopped
- ½ red onion, finely chopped
- 1 cherry pepper, seeded and finely chopped
- ¼ cup extra-virgin olive oil
- 2 tablespoons white wine vinegar
- 1 teaspoon chopped fresh basil
- 1 garlic clove, minced
- Salt
- Freshly ground black pepper

DIRECTIONS:

1. Cook the whole grains according to package directions. Allow to cool. In a large bowl, toss the grains, chickpeas, spinach, cucumber, bell pepper, fennel, celery, carrot, tomato, red onion, and cherry pepper.

2. In a small bowl, whisk together the olive oil, vinegar, basil, and garlic. Season with salt and pepper. Toss with the salad and serve.

NUTRITION: Calories: 401 Fat: 18g Protein: 12g Carbohydrates: 50g

15. Green Bean and Potato Salad

Preparation time: 15 minutes

Cooking time: 15 minutes

Servings: 4

INGREDIENTS:

- 2 russet potatoes, peeled and cut into 1-inch pieces

- 2 cups green beans, trimmed
- ¼ cup extra-virgin olive oil
- Juice of ½ lemon
- 1 teaspoon Italian Herb Blend
- 1 teaspoon salt
- ½ teaspoon freshly ground black pepper

DIRECTIONS:

1. Put the potatoes in a saucepan, cover with water, and bring to a boil over high heat. Cook for about 10 minutes, until tender. Drain and set aside to cool.

2. While the potatoes are cooling, fill the same saucepan with water and bring to a boil over high heat. Fill a large bowl with ice cubes and cold water.

3. Add the green beans to the boiling water and blanch for about 3 minutes, then remove with tongs or a sieve and immediately plunge them into the ice bath. Once cool, drain.

4. Combine the potatoes and green beans in a large bowl. Drizzle the olive oil over the vegetables and squeeze in the lemon juice. Add the Italian herb blend, salt, and pepper and toss to combine.

NUTRITION: Calories: 282 Fat: 14g Protein: 5g Carbohydrates: 37g

16. Shrimp Salad

Preparation time: 15 minutes

Cooking time: 5 minutes

Servings: 4

INGREDIENTS:

- 1-pound large shrimp, peeled and deveined
- Juice of ½ lemon
- 2 celery stalks, chopped
- 3 scallions, chopped
- 1 garlic clove, minced
- Salt
- Freshly ground black pepper
- ½ cup vegan mayonnaise

DIRECTIONS:

1. Put the shrimp in a skillet and add a few tablespoons of water. Cook over medium heat for 2 to 3 minutes, until the shrimp turn pink. Drain and pat dry. Cut the shrimp into bite-size pieces and transfer a bowl.

2. Add the lemon juice and toss, then add the celery, scallions, and garlic. Season with salt and pepper. Toss again to combine. Add the vegan mayonnaise and fold gently to combine.

NUTRITION: Calories: 185 Fat: 11g Protein: 18g Carbohydrates: 4g

17. Warm Potato Salad

Preparation time: 15 minutes

Cooking time: 10 minutes

Servings: 4

INGREDIENTS:

- 6 red potatoes, cut into 1-inch pieces

- 1 tablespoon white wine vinegar
- 3 large eggs, hard-boiled, peeled, and chopped
- 2 celery stalks, finely chopped
- 1 small onion, finely chopped
- ½ cup mayonnaise or vegan mayonnaise
- 1 teaspoon Dijon mustard
- 1 teaspoon salt
- ¼ teaspoon freshly ground black pepper

DIRECTIONS:

1. Put the potatoes in a saucepan, cover with water, and bring to a boil over high heat. Cook for about 10 minutes, until tender. Drain and transfer to a large bowl, then sprinkle with the vinegar.

2. Add the eggs, celery, and onion and toss. Add the mayonnaise, mustard, salt, and pepper and toss to combine. Serve.

NUTRITION: Calories: 474 Fat: 25g Protein: 11g Carbohydrates: 53g

18. Summer Rainbow Salad

Preparation time: 15 minutes

Cooking time: 0 minutes

Servings: 4

INGREDIENTS:

- 1 cup chopped red or green leaf lettuce
- 1 cup chopped iceberg lettuce
- ½ cup baby arugula

- ½ cup chopped radicchio
- 1 cup mixed chopped or sliced vegetables, such as red cabbage, red onion, radish, red or yellow tomato, carrot, cucumber, and/or avocado
- ¼ cup extra-virgin olive oil
- Juice of ½ lemon
- ½ teaspoon salt
- ¼ teaspoon freshly ground black pepper
- ¼ teaspoon dried oregano

DIRECTIONS:

1. In a large salad bowl, combine the lettuces, arugula, radicchio, and mixed vegetables and gently toss.
2. In a small bowl, whisk together the olive oil, lemon juice, salt, pepper, and oregano. Pour the dressing over the salad and toss well to coat.

NUTRITION: Calories: 137 Fat: 14g Protein: 1g Carbohydrates: 4g

19. Arugula and White Bean Salad

Preparation time: 15 minutes

Cooking time: 0 minutes

Servings: 2

INGREDIENTS:

- 1 (15-ounce) can cannellini beans, rinsed and drained
- 2 cups baby arugula
- ¼ cup extra-virgin olive oil

- Juice of ½ lemon
- ½ teaspoon dried oregano
- ½ teaspoon salt
- ¼ teaspoon freshly ground black pepper
- 4 Italian seeded bread slices, toasted

DIRECTIONS:

1. In a medium bowl, combine the beans and arugula. In a small bowl, whisk together the olive oil, lemon juice, oregano, salt, and pepper. Pour over the salad and toss to coat.

2. To serve, spoon heaping portions of the salad over the toast.

NUTRITION: Calories: 469 Fat: 29g Protein: 14g Carbohydrates: 42g

20. Fennel and Orange Salad

Preparation time: 15 minutes

Cooking time: 0 minutes

Servings: 6

INGREDIENTS:

- 4 navel oranges, peeled, halved, and thinly sliced
- 3 fennel bulbs, trimmed and thinly sliced, fronds reserved for garnish
- 2 tablespoons extra-virgin olive oil
- 1 tablespoon white wine vinegar
- Salt
- Freshly ground black pepper

DIRECTIONS:

1. In a large bowl, combine the orange and fennel slices. In a small bowl, whisk together the olive oil and vinegar. Season with salt and pepper.

2. Pour the dressing over the orange and fennel and toss to combine. Roughly chop the fennel fronds and sprinkle them on top.

NUTRITION: Calories: 122 Fat: 5g Protein: 2g Carbohydrates: 20g

SOUP RECIPES

21. Summer Berry Soup

Preparation time: 15 minutes

Cooking time: 10 minutes

Servings: 4

INGREDIENTS:

- ½ cup apple juice
- ¼ cup strawberries
- ¼ cup raspberries
- ¼ cup blackberries
- ¼ cup blueberries
- 1 teaspoon potato starch
- ¼ teaspoon ground cinnamon

DIRECTIONS:

1. In the saucepan, pour in the apple juice. Add all the berries and cinnamon from the field. Cover the lid and cook the ingredients.
2. In a bottle, apply three tablespoons of apple juice mixture, apply potato starch, and whisk until smooth.
3. Then pour the berry soup into the starch mixture and stir until the soup is thickened. Cover the lid and leave the soup for 10 minutes to recover.

NUTRITION: Calories 71 Protein 0.8g Carbohydrates 17.3g Fat 0.4g

22. **Green Beans Soup**

Preparation time: 15 minutes

Cooking time: 40 minutes

Servings: 4

INGREDIENTS:

- ½ onion, diced
- 1/3 cup green beans, soaked
- 3 cups of water
- ½ sweet pepper, chopped
- 2 potatoes, chopped
- 1 tablespoon fresh cilantro, chopped
- 1 teaspoon chili flakes

DIRECTIONS:

1. In the saucepan, put all the ingredients and close the lid. On medium heat, cook the soup for 40 minutes or until the ingredients are all tender.

NUTRITION: Calories 87 Protein 2.3g Carbohydrates 19.8g Fat 0.2g

23. **Turkey Soup**

Preparation time: 15 minutes

Cooking time: 22 minutes

Servings: 4

INGREDIENTS:

- 1 potato, diced

- 1 cup ground turkey
- 1 teaspoon cayenne pepper
- 1 onion, diced
- 1 tablespoon olive oil
- ¼ carrot, diced
- 2 cups of water

DIRECTIONS:

1. In a saucepan, heat the olive oil and add the diced onion and carrot. For 3 minutes, prepare the vegetables. Then stir them well and add the cayenne pepper and ground turkey.

2. Attach the diced potato and stir well with the spices. Cook them for an extra 2 minutes. Add water, too.

3. Check if all the ingredients have been put in. Cover the lid and simmer for 20 minutes to make the broth.

NUTRITION: Calories 317 Protein 31.8g Carbohydrates 14.2g Fat 16.9g

24. Beef Soup

Preparation time: 15 minutes

Cooking time: 44 minutes

Servings: 4

INGREDIENTS:

- 1-pound beef sirloin, chopped
- 4 oz. leek, chopped
- 1 tablespoon margarine

- 1 teaspoon chili powder
- 1 potato, chopped
- 3 cups of water

DIRECTIONS:

1. In the saucepan, toss and heat the margarine. Then add the sliced sirloin of beef, chili powder, and leek. Cook the ingredients for 4 minutes on each.
2. Include the diced potato and water after this. Get the cover closed. On medium heat, prepare the beef broth for 40 minutes.

NUTRITION: Calories 288 Protein 35.8g Carbohydrates 11.8g Fat 10.2g

25. Asparagus Cream Soup

Preparation time: 15 minutes

Cooking time: 30 minutes

Servings: 4

INGREDIENTS:

- 2 cups low-sodium chicken stock
- 1 cup asparagus, chopped
- 2 tablespoons low-fat sour cream
- 1 teaspoon dried oregano
- 1 garlic clove, diced
- 1 teaspoon olive oil
- 1 cup broccoli, chopped

DIRECTIONS:

1. In a saucepan, add in the olive oil and boil it for 1 minute. Attach the garlic and roast it for another 1 minute. Add all the remaining ingredients from the list above and close the lid after that.

2. For 25 minutes, boil the broth. Then mix the soup until smooth with the aid of the immersion blender. Simmer the broth for an additional 3 minutes.

NUTRITION: Calories 38 Protein 2.2g Carbohydrates 4.1g Fat 1.8g

26. Pasta Soup

Preparation time: 15 minutes

Cooking time: 13 minutes

Servings: 4

INGREDIENTS:

- 2 oz. whole-grain pasta
- ½ cup corn kernels
- 1 oz. carrot, shredded
- 3 oz. celery stalk, chopped
- 2 cups low-sodium chicken stock
- 1 teaspoon ground black pepper

DIRECTIONS:

1. Bring the chicken stock to boil and add shredded carrot and celery stalk. Simmer the liquid for 5 minutes.

2. After this, add corn kernels, ground black pepper, and pasta. Stir the soup well. Simmer it on the medium heat for 8 minutes.

NUTRITION: Calories 263 Protein 11.8g Carbohydrates 49.6g Fat 2.6g

27. Black Beans Soup

Preparation time: 15 minutes

Cooking time: 21 minutes

Servings: 4

INGREDIENTS:

- 2 cups black beans, cooked
- 1 yellow onion, diced
- ¼ cup sweet pepper, chopped
- 5 cups low-sodium chicken broth
- 1 carrot, shredded
- 1 teaspoon dried oregano
- ½ teaspoon ground cumin
- 1 teaspoon chili flakes
- ½ cup fresh cilantro, chopped
- 1 tablespoon avocado oil

DIRECTIONS:

1. Pour avocado oil in the saucepan and add shredded carrot and onion. Cook the vegetables for 4 minutes. Stir them from time to time.

2. After this, add sweet pepper, black beans, oregano, and all the remaining ingredients. Close the lid and cook the soup on medium heat for 15 minutes.

3. After this, blend the soup for 1 minute with the help of the immersion blender. The cooked soup should be smooth. Simmer it for 1 minute more. Serve.

NUTRITION: Calories 251 Protein 16.1g Carbohydrates 44.7g Fat 1.3g

28. Cucumber and Melon Soup

Preparation time: 15 minutes

Cooking time: 0 minutes

Servings: 4

INGREDIENTS:

- 4 cucumbers, chopped
- 9 oz. melon, chopped
- ½ cup fresh cilantro, chopped
- 1 teaspoon honey
- 2 tablespoons lemon juice
- ½ teaspoon cayenne pepper

DIRECTIONS:

1. Put all ingredients in the blender and blend until smooth. Transfer the smooth soup to the serving bowls and refrigerate for 15 minutes before serving.

NUTRITION: Calories 75 Protein 2.6g Carbohydrates 17.9g Fat 0.6g

29. Wild Rice Soup

Preparation time: 15 minutes

Cooking time: 30 minutes

Servings: 4

INGREDIENTS:

- ¼ cup wild rice
- 2 cups low-sodium chicken broth
- 1 potato, chopped
- 1 teaspoon ground turmeric
- ¼ teaspoon dried dill
- 1 tablespoon low-fat sour cream

DIRECTIONS:

1. In a saucepan, add in the chicken broth and bring it to a boil. Drizzle with wild rice and simmer for 10 minutes.
2. Add the potato, turmeric, dill, and low-fat sour cream after that. For 20 minutes, close the lid and prepare the broth.

NUTRITION: Calories 171 Protein 7.3g Carbohydrates 32.6g Fat 1.4g

30. Green Detox Soup

Preparation time: 15 minutes

Cooking time: 12 minutes

Servings: 4

INGREDIENTS:

- 1 onion, diced
- 1 large zucchini, chopped
- 1 teaspoon fresh mint, chopped
- ½ cup celery stalk, chopped

- 1 teaspoon ground paprika

- 1 tablespoon olive oil

- 2 tablespoons lime juice

- 1 cup low-fat yogurt

DIRECTIONS:

1. Heat olive oil in the saucepan. Add diced onion and cook it for 2 minutes. Stir it well. Add zucchini, mint, and celery stalk. Cook the vegetables for 10 minutes. Stir them from time to time.

2. After this, add lime juice and ground paprika. Blend the vegetables with the help of the immersion blender and remove them from the heat. Add yogurt and stir the soup well.

NUTRITION: Calories 103 Protein 5g Carbohydrates 10.8g Fat 4.5g

SIDE RECIPES

31. Basmati Rice

Preparation time: 7 minutes

Cooking time: 20 minutes

Servings: 4

INGREDIENTS:

- 1 cup basmati rice
- 2 tablespoons olive oil
- 1 teaspoon salt
- 2 ½ cup chicken stock

DIRECTIONS:

1. Pour olive oil in the pan and heat it up. Add basmati rice and roast it for 3 minutes. Stir it from time to time. Then add salt and chicken stock.
2. Mix up the ingredients until homogenous. Close the lid and boil rice for 15 minutes or until it soaks all the liquid.

NUTRITION: Calories 235 Fat 7.7g Carbs 37.4g Protein 3.7g

32. Spiced Buckwheat

Preparation time: 10 minutes

Cooking time: 25 minutes

Servings: 4

INGREDIENTS:

- ½ teaspoon ground cardamom
- ¾ teaspoon ground cinnamon
- ¾ teaspoon ground ginger
- 1 teaspoon salt
- 2 tablespoons butter
- 1 tablespoon olive oil
- 1 ½ cup buckwheat
- 3 cups beef broth

DIRECTIONS:

1. Place olive oil in the pan and heat it up. Add buckwheat and butter. Roast the buckwheat for 5 minutes over the medium heat. Stir it from time to time.

2. Then add ground cardamom, ground cinnamon, salt, and ginger. Mix up the buckwheat. Add beef broth, mix up, and cook buckwheat for 20 minutes over the low heat. Serve.

NUTRITION: Calories 331 Fat 12.5g Carbs 47g Protein 12.2g

33. Coconut Bulgur

Preparation time: 7 minutes

Cooking time: 20 minutes

Servings: 2

INGREDIENTS:

- ½ cup bulgur
- 1 teaspoon tomato paste

- ½ white onion, diced
- 2 tablespoons coconut oil
- 1 ½ cup chicken stock

DIRECTIONS:

1. Toss coconut oil in the pan and melt it. Add diced onion and roast it until light brown. Then add bulgur and stir well. Cook bulgur in coconut oil for 3 minutes.

2. Then add tomato paste and mix up bulgur until homogenous. Add chicken stock. Close the lid and cook bulgur for 15 minutes over the medium heat. The cooked bulgur should soak all liquid.

NUTRITION: Calories 257 Fat 14.5g Carbs 30.2g Protein 5.2g

34. Cardamom Couscous

Preparation time: 10 minutes

Cooking time: 10 minutes

Servings: 4

INGREDIENTS:

- 1 cup yellow couscous
- ½ teaspoon ground cardamom
- 1 cup chicken stock
- 1 tablespoon butter
- 1 teaspoon salt
- ½ teaspoon red pepper

DIRECTIONS:

1. Toss butter in the pan and melt it. Add couscous and roast it for 1 minute over the high heat. Then add ground cardamom, salt, and red pepper. Stir it well.
2. Add chicken stock and bring the mixture to boil. Simmer couscous for 5 minutes with the closed lid.

NUTRITION: Calories 196 Fat 3.4g Carbs 35g Protein 5.9g

35. <u>Parmesan Polenta</u>

Preparation time: 8 minutes

Cooking time: 45 minutes

Servings: 4

INGREDIENTS:

- 1 cup polenta
- 1 ½ cup water
- 2 cups chicken stock
- ½ cup cream
- 1/3 cup Parmesan, grated

DIRECTIONS:

1. Put polenta in the pot. Add water, chicken stock, cream, and Parmesan. Mix up polenta well. Then preheat oven to 355F.
2. Cook polenta in the oven for 45 minutes. Mix up the cooked meal with the help of the spoon carefully before serving.

NUTRITION: Calories 208 Fat 5.3g Carbs 32.2g Protein 8g

36. Buttery Millet

Preparation time: 10 minutes

Cooking time: 15 minutes

Servings: 3

INGREDIENTS:

- ¼ cup mushrooms, sliced
- ¾ cup onion, diced
- 1 tablespoon olive oil
- 1 teaspoon salt
- 3 tablespoons milk
- ½ cup millet
- 1 cup of water
- 1 teaspoon butter

DIRECTIONS:

1. Pour olive oil in the skillet and add the onion. Add mushrooms and roast the vegetables for 10 minutes over the medium heat. Stir them from time to time.
2. Meanwhile, pour water in the pan. Add millet and salt. Cook the millet with the closed lid for 15 minutes over the medium heat.
3. Then add the cooked mushroom mixture in the millet. Add milk and butter. Mix up the millet well.

NUTRITION: Calories 198 Fat 7.7g Carbs 27.9g Protein 4.7g

37. Cayenne Barley

Preparation time: 7 minutes

Cooking time: 42 minutes

Servings: 5

INGREDIENTS:

- 1 cup barley
- 3 cups chicken stock
- ½ teaspoon cayenne pepper
- 1 teaspoon salt
- ½ teaspoon chili pepper
- ½ teaspoon ground black pepper
- 1 teaspoon butter
- 1 teaspoon olive oil

DIRECTIONS:

1. Place barley and olive oil in the pan. Roast barley on high heat for 1 minute. Stir it well. Then add salt, chili pepper, ground black pepper, cayenne pepper, and butter.
2. Add chicken stock. Close the lid and cook barley for 40 minutes over the medium-low heat.

NUTRITION: Calories 152 Fat 2.9g Carbs 27.8g Protein 5.1g

38. Dill Farro

Preparation time: 8 minutes

Cooking time: 40 minutes

Servings: 4

INGREDIENTS:

- 1 cup farro

- 3 cups beef broth
- 1 teaspoon salt
- 1 tablespoon almond butter
- 1 tablespoon dried dill

DIRECTIONS:

1. Place farro in the pan. Add beef broth, dried dill, and salt. Close the lid and bring the mixture to boil. Then boil it for 35 minutes over the medium-low heat.
2. When the time is over, open the lid and add almond butter. Mix up the cooked farro well.

NUTRITION: Calories 95 Fat 3.3g Carbs 10.1g Protein 6.4g

39. Wheatberry and Walnuts Salad

Preparation time: 10 minutes

Cooking time: 50 minutes

Servings: 2

INGREDIENTS:

- ¼ cup of wheat berries
- 1 cup of water
- 1 teaspoon salt
- 2 tablespoons walnuts, chopped
- 1 tablespoon chives, chopped
- ¼ cup fresh parsley, chopped
- 2 oz pomegranate seeds
- 1 tablespoon canola oil

- 1 teaspoon chili flakes

DIRECTIONS:

1. Place wheat berries and water in the pan. Add salt and simmer the ingredients for 50 minutes over the medium heat.

2. Meanwhile, mix up together walnuts, chives, parsley, pomegranate seeds, and chili flakes. When the wheatberry is cooked, transfer it in the walnut mixture. Add canola oil and mix up the salad well.

NUTRITION: Calories 160 Fat 11.8g Carbs 12g Protein 3.4g

40. Curry Rice

Preparation time: 10 minutes

Cooking time: 1 hour 15 minutes

Servings: 5

INGREDIENTS:

- 1 tablespoon curry paste
- ¼ cup milk
- 1 cup wheatberries
- ½ cup of rice
- 1 teaspoon salt
- 4 tablespoons olive oil
- 6 cups chicken stock

DIRECTIONS:

1. Place wheatberries and chicken stock in the pan. Close the lid and cook the mixture for 1 hour over the medium heat. Then add rice, olive oil, and salt. Stir well.

2. Mix up together milk and curry paste. Add the curry liquid in the rice-wheatberry mixture and stir well. Boil the meal for 15 minutes with the closed lid. When the rice is cooked, all the meal is cooked.

NUTRITION: Calories 232 Fat 15g Carbs 23.5g Protein 3.9g

MAIN RECIPES: SEAFOOD

41. Easy Breaded Shrimp

Preparation time: 15 minutes

Cooking time: 4-6 minutes

Servings: 4

INGREDIENTS:

- 2 large eggs
- 1 tablespoon water
- 2 cups seasoned Italian bread crumbs
- 1 teaspoon salt
- 1 cup flour
- 1 pound (454 g) large shrimp (21 to 25), peeled and deveined
- Extra-virgin olive oil, as needed

DIRECTIONS:

1. In a small bowl, beat the eggs with the water, then transfer to a shallow dish. Add the bread crumbs and salt to a separate shallow dish, then mix well. Place the flour into a third shallow dish.

2. Coat the shrimp in the flour, then the beaten egg, and finally the bread crumbs. Place on a plate and repeat with all of the shrimp.

3. Heat a skillet over high heat. Pour in enough olive oil to coat the bottom of the skillet. Cook the shrimp in the hot skillet for 2 to

3 minutes on each side. Remove and drain on a paper towel. Serve warm.

NUTRITION: Calories: 714 Fat: 34.0g Protein: 37.0g Carbs: 63.0g

42. Pesto Shrimp over Zoodles

Preparation time: 15 minutes

Cooking time: 10 minutes

Servings: 4

INGREDIENTS:

- 1 pound (454 g) fresh shrimp, peeled and deveined
- Salt and freshly ground black pepper, to taste
- 2 tablespoons extra-virgin olive oil
- ½ small onion, slivered
- 8 ounces (227 g) store-bought jarred pesto
- ¾ cup crumbled goat or feta cheese, plus additional for serving
- 2 large zucchinis, spiralized, for serving
- ¼ cup chopped flat-leaf Italian parsley, for garnish

DIRECTIONS:

1. In a bowl, season the shrimp with salt and pepper. Set aside. In a large skillet, heat the olive oil over medium-high heat. Sauté the onion until just golden, 5 to 6 minutes.

2. Reduce the heat to low and add the pesto and cheese, whisking to combine and melt the cheese. Bring to a low simmer and add the shrimp.

3. Reduce the heat back to low and cover. Cook until the shrimp is cooked through and pink, about 3 to 4 minutes.

4. Serve the shrimp warm over zoodles, garnishing with chopped parsley and additional crumbled cheese.

NUTRITION: Calories: 491 Fat: 35.0g Protein: 29.0g Carbs: 15.0g

43. <u>Salt and Pepper Calamari and Scallops</u>

Preparation time: 15 minutes

Cooking time: 10 minutes

Servings: 4

INGREDIENTS:

- 8 ounces (227 g) calamari steaks, cut into ½-inch-thick rings
- 8 ounces (227 g) sea scallops
- 1½ teaspoons salt, divided
- 1 teaspoon garlic powder
- 1 teaspoon freshly ground black pepper
- 1/3 cup extra-virgin olive oil
- 2 tablespoons almond butter

DIRECTIONS:

1. Place the calamari and scallops on several layers of paper towels and pat dry. Sprinkle with 1 teaspoon of salt and allow to sit for 15 minutes at room temperature.

2. Pat dry with additional paper towels. Sprinkle with pepper and garlic powder. In a deep medium skillet, heat the olive oil and butter over medium-high heat.

3. When the oil is hot but not smoking, add the scallops and calamari in a single layer to the skillet and sprinkle with the remaining ½ teaspoon of salt.

4. Cook for 2 to 4 minutes on each side, depending on the size of the scallops, until just golden but still slightly opaque in center.

5. Using a slotted spoon, remove from the skillet and transfer to a serving platter. Allow the cooking oil to cool slightly and drizzle over the seafood before serving.

NUTRITION: Calories: 309 Fat: 25.0g Protein: 18.0g Carbs: 3.0g

44. Grilled Fish on Lemons

Preparation Time: 10 minutes

Cooking Time: 10 minutes

Servings: 4

INGREDIENTS:

- 4 (4-ounce) fish fillets
- Nonstick cooking spray
- 3 to 4 medium lemons
- 1 tablespoon extra-virgin olive oil
- ¼ teaspoon freshly ground black pepper
- ¼ teaspoon kosher or sea salt

DIRECTIONS:

1. Using paper towels, pat the fillets dry and let stand at room temperature for 10 minutes.

2. Meanwhile, coat the cold cooking grate of the grill with nonstick cooking spray, and preheat the grill to 400°F, or medium-high heat. Or preheat a grill pan over medium-high heat on the stovetop.

3. Cut one lemon in half and set half aside. Slice the remaining half of that lemon and the remaining lemons into ¼-inch-thick slices. You should have about 12 to 16 lemon slices.

4. In a small bowl, squeeze 1 tablespoon of juice out of the reserved lemon half. Add the oil to the bowl with the lemon juice and mix well.

5. Brush both sides of the fish with the oil mixture, and sprinkle evenly with pepper and salt.

6. Carefully place the lemon slices on the grill (or the grill pan), arranging 3 to 4 slices together in the shape of a fish fillet, and repeat with the remaining slices.

7. Place the fish fillets directly on top of the lemon slices, and grill with the lid closed. If you're grilling on the stovetop, cover with a large pot lid or aluminum foil.

8. Turn the fish halfway through the cooking time only if the fillets are more than half an inch thick. The fish is done and ready to serve when it just begins to separate into flakes (chunks) when pressed gently with a fork.

NUTRITION: Calories: 147 Fat: 5g Carbs: 1g Protein: 22g

45. Vinegar Honeyed Salmon

Preparation Time: 10 minutes

Cooking Time: 5 minutes

Servings: 4

INGREDIENTS:

- 4 (8-ounce) salmon fillets
- 1/2 cup balsamic vinegar
- 1 tablespoon honey
- Black pepper (ground) and sea salt, to taste
- 1 tablespoon olive oil

DIRECTIONS:

1. In a mixing bowl, add honey and vinegar. Mix together well. Season fish fillets with the black pepper (ground) and sea salt; brush with honey glaze.

2. Take a medium saucepan or skillet, add oil. Heat over medium heat. Add salmon fillets and stir-cook until medium-rare in the center and lightly browned for 3-4 minutes per side. Serve warm.

NUTRITION: Calories: 481 Fat: 16g Carbohydrates: 24gProtein: 1.5g

46. Orange Fish Meal

Preparation Time: 10 minutes

Cooking Time: 5 minutes

Servings: 4

INGREDIENTS:

- ¼ teaspoon kosher or sea salt

- 1 tablespoon extra-virgin olive oil

- 1 tablespoon orange juice

- 4 (4-ounce) tilapia fillets, with or without skin

- ¼ cup chopped red onion

- 1 avocado, pitted, skinned, and sliced

DIRECTIONS:

1. Take a baking dish of 9-inch; add olive oil, orange juice, and salt. Mix well. Add fish fillets and coat well. Add onions over fish fillets.

2. Cover with plastic wrap. Microwave for 3 minutes until fish is cooked well and easy to flake. Serve warm with sliced avocado on top.

NUTRITION: Calories: 231 Fat: 9g Carbohydrates: 8g Protein: 2.5g

47. Shrimp Zoodles

Preparation Time: 10 minutes

Cooking Time: 5 minutes

Servings: 2

INGREDIENTS:

- 2 tablespoons chopped parsley

- 2 teaspoons minced garlic

- 1 teaspoon salt

- ½ teaspoon black pepper

- 2 medium zucchinis, spiralized

- 3/4 pounds medium shrimp, peeled & deveined

- 1 tablespoon olive oil
- 1 lemon, juiced and zested

DIRECTIONS:

1. Take a medium saucepan or skillet, add oil, lemon juice, and lemon zest. Heat over a medium heat. Add shrimps and stir-cook 1 minute per side. Add garlic and red pepper flakes; cook for 1 more minute.

2. Add zoodles and stir gently; cook for 3 minutes until cooked to satisfaction. Season with salt and black pepper and serve warm with parsley on top.

NUTRITION: Calories: 329 Fat: 12g Carbohydrates: 11g Protein: 25g

48. Tuna Nutty Salad

Preparation Time: 10 minutes

Cooking Time: 0 minute

Servings: 4

INGREDIENTS:

- 1 tablespoon chopped tarragon
- 1 stalk celery, trimmed and finely diced
- 1 medium shallot, diced
- 3 tablespoons chopped chives
- 1 (5-ounce) can tuna (covered in olive oil) drained and flaked
- 1 teaspoon Dijon mustard
- 2-3 tablespoons mayonnaise
- 1/4 teaspoon salt

- 1/8 teaspoon pepper
- 1/4 cup pine nuts, toasted

DIRECTIONS:

1. In a large salad bowl, add tuna, shallot, chives, tarragon, and celery. Combine to mix well with each other.

2. In a mixing bowl, add mayonnaise, mustard, salt, and black pepper. Combine to mix well with each other.

3. Add mayonnaise mixture to a salad bowl; toss well to combine. Add pine nuts and toss again. Serve fresh.

NUTRITION: Calories: 236 Fat: 14g Carbohydrates: 4g Protein: 20g

49. Salmon Skillet Supper

Preparation Time: 15 minutes

Cooking Time: 15 minutes

Servings: 4

INGREDIENTS:

- 1 tablespoon extra-virgin olive oil
- 2 garlic cloves minced
- 1 teaspoon smoked paprika
- 1-pint grape or cherry tomatoes, quartered
- 1 (12-ounce) jar roasted red peppers
- 1 tablespoon water
- ¼ teaspoon freshly ground black pepper
- ¼ teaspoon kosher or sea salt
- 1-pound salmon fillets, skin removed, cut into 8 pieces

- 1 tablespoon freshly squeezed lemon juice (from ½ medium lemon)

DIRECTIONS:

1. In a large skillet over medium heat, heat the oil. Add the garlic and smoked paprika and cook for 1 minute, stirring often. Add the tomatoes, roasted peppers, water, black pepper, and salt.

2. Turn up the heat to medium-high, bring to a simmer, and cook for 3 minutes, stirring occasionally and smashing the tomatoes with a wooden spoon toward the end of the cooking time.

3. Add the salmon to the skillet, and spoon some of the sauce over the top. Cover and cook for 10 to 12 minutes, or until the salmon is cooked through (145°F using a meat thermometer) and just starts to flake.

4. Remove the skillet from the heat, and drizzle lemon juice over the top of the fish. Stir the sauce, then break up the salmon into chunks with a fork. You can serve it straight from the skillet.

NUTRITION: Calories: 289 Fat: 13g Carbs: 17gProtein: 31g

50. Weeknight Sheet Pan Fish Dinner

Preparation Time: 10 minutes

Cooking Time: 10 minutes

Servings: 4

INGREDIENTS:

- Nonstick cooking spray
- 2 tablespoons extra-virgin olive oil
- 1 tablespoon balsamic vinegar

- 4 (4-ounce) fish fillets (½ inch thick)
- 2½ cups green beans
- 1-pint cherry or grape tomatoes

DIRECTIONS:

1. Preheat the oven to 400°F. Coat two large, rimmed baking sheets with nonstick cooking spray. In a small bowl, whisk together the oil and vinegar. Set aside. Place two pieces of fish on each baking sheet.

2. In a large bowl, combine the beans and tomatoes. Pour in the oil and vinegar and toss gently to coat.

3. Pour half of the green bean mixture over the fish on one baking sheet, and the remaining half over the fish on the other.

4. Turn the fish over and rub it in the oil mixture to coat. Spread the vegetables evenly on the baking sheets so hot air can circulate around them.

5. Bake for 5 to 8 minutes, until the fish is just opaque and not translucent. The fish is done and ready to serve when it just begins to separate into flakes (chunks) when pressed gently with a fork.

NUTRITION: Calories: 193 Fat: 8g Carbs: 42g Protein: 23g

51. Crispy Polenta Fish Sticks

Preparation Time: 15 minutes

Cooking Time: 10 minutes

Servings: 4

INGREDIENTS:

- 2 large eggs, lightly beaten
- 1 tablespoon 2% milk
- 1-pound skinned fish fillets sliced into 20 (1-inchwide) strips
- ½ cup yellow cornmeal
- ½ cup whole-wheat panko breadcrumbs
- ¼ teaspoon smoked paprika
- ¼ teaspoon kosher or sea salt
- ¼ teaspoon freshly ground black pepper
- Nonstick cooking spray

DIRECTIONS:

1. Place a large, rimmed baking sheet in the oven. Preheat the oven to 400°F with the pan inside. In a large bowl, mix the eggs and milk. Using a fork, add the fish strips to the egg mixture and stir gently to coat.

2. Put the cornmeal, breadcrumbs, smoked paprika, salt, and pepper in a quart-size zip-top plastic bag.

3. Using a fork or tongs, transfer the fish to the bag, letting the excess egg drip off into the bowl before transferring. Seal the bag and shake gently to completely coat each fish stick.

4. With oven mitts, carefully remove the hot baking sheet from the oven and spray it with nonstick cooking spray.

5. Using a fork or tongs, remove the fish sticks from the bag and arrange them on the hot baking sheet, with space between them so the hot air can circulate and crisp them up.

6. Bake for 5 to 8 minutes, until gentle pressure with a fork causes the fish to flake, then serve.

NUTRITION: Calories: 256 Fat: 6g Carbs: 20g Protein: 29g

MAIN RECIPES: POULTRY

52. Creamy Chicken Breasts

Preparation Time: 10 minutes

Cooking Time: 12 minutes

Servings: 4

INGREDIENTS:

- 4 chicken breasts, skinless and boneless
- 1 tbsp basil pesto
- 1 1/2 tbsp cornstarch
- 1/4 cup roasted red peppers, chopped
- 1/3 cup heavy cream
- 1 tsp Italian seasoning
- 1 tsp garlic, minced
- 1 cup chicken broth
- Pepper
- Salt

DIRECTIONS:

1. Add chicken into the instant pot. Season chicken with Italian seasoning, pepper, and salt. Sprinkle with garlic. Pour broth over chicken. Seal pot with lid and cook on high for 8 minutes.

2. Once done, allow to release pressure naturally for 5 minutes then release remaining using quick release. Remove lid. Transfer chicken on a plate and clean the instant pot.

3. Set instant pot on sauté mode. Add heavy cream, pesto, cornstarch, and red pepper to the pot and stir well and cook for 3-4 minutes.

4. Return chicken to the pot and coat well with the sauce. Serve and enjoy.

NUTRITION: Calories 341 Fat 15.2 g Carbohydrates 4.4 g Protein 43.8 g

53. Cheese Garlic Chicken & Potatoes

Preparation Time: 10 minutes

Cooking Time: 13 minutes

Servings: 4

INGREDIENTS:

- 2 lb. chicken breasts, skinless, boneless, cut into chunks
- 1 tbsp olive oil
- 3/4 cup chicken broth
- 1 tbsp Italian seasoning
- 1 tbsp garlic powder
- 1 tsp garlic, minced
- 1 1/2 cup parmesan cheese, shredded
- 1 lb. potatoes, chopped
- Pepper

- Salt

DIRECTIONS:

1. Add oil into the inner pot of instant pot and set the pot on sauté mode. Add chicken and cook until browned. Add remaining ingredients except for cheese and stir well.

2. Seal pot with lid and cook on high for 8 minutes. Once done, release pressure using quick release. Remove lid. Top with cheese and cover with lid for 5 minutes or until cheese is melted. Serve and enjoy.

NUTRITION: Calories 674 Fat 29 g Carbohydrates 21.4 g Protein 79.7 g

54. Easy Chicken Scampi

Preparation Time: 10 minutes

Cooking Time: 25 minutes

Servings: 4

INGREDIENTS:

- 3 chicken breasts, skinless, boneless, and sliced
- 1 tsp garlic, minced
- 1 tbsp Italian seasoning
- 2 cups chicken broth
- 1 bell pepper, sliced
- 1/2 onion, sliced
- Pepper
- Salt

DIRECTIONS:

1. Add chicken into the instant pot and top with remaining ingredients. Seal pot with lid and cook on high for 25 minutes. Once done, release pressure using quick release. Remove lid.

2. Remove chicken from pot and shred using a fork. Return shredded chicken to the pot and stir well. Serve over cooked whole grain pasta and top with cheese.

NUTRITION: Calories 254 Fat 9.9 g Carbohydrates 4.6 g Protein 34.6 g

55. Protein Packed Chicken Bean Rice

Preparation Time: 10 minutes

Cooking Time: 15 minutes

Servings: 6

INGREDIENTS:

- 1 lb. chicken breasts, skinless, boneless, and cut into chunks
- 14 oz can cannellini beans, rinsed and drained
- 4 cups chicken broth
- 2 cups brown rice
- 1 tbsp Italian seasoning
- 1 small onion, chopped
- 1 tbsp garlic, chopped
- 1 tbsp olive oil
- Pepper
- Salt

DIRECTIONS:

1. Add oil into the inner pot of instant pot and set the pot on sauté mode. Add garlic and onion and sauté for 3 minutes. Add remaining ingredients and stir everything well.

2. Seal pot with a lid and select manual and set timer for 12 minutes. Once done, release pressure using quick release. Remove lid. Stir well and serve.

NUTRITION: Calories 494 Fat 11.3 g Carbohydrates 61.4 g Protein 34.2 g

56. Pesto Vegetable Chicken

Preparation Time: 10 minutes

Cooking Time: 25 minutes

Servings: 4

INGREDIENTS:

- 1 1/2 lb. chicken thighs, skinless, boneless, and cut into pieces
- 1/2 cup chicken broth
- 1/4 cup fresh parsley, chopped
- 2 cups cherry tomatoes, halved
- 1 cup basil pesto
- 3/4 lb. asparagus, trimmed and cut in half
- 2/3 cup sun-dried tomatoes, drained and chopped
- 2 tbsp olive oil
- Pepper
- Salt

DIRECTIONS:

1. Add oil into the inner pot of instant pot and set the pot on sauté mode. Add chicken and sauté for 5 minutes. Add remaining ingredients except for tomatoes and stir well.

2. Seal pot with a lid and select manual and set timer for 15 minutes. Once done, release pressure using quick release. Remove lid.

3. Add tomatoes and stir well. Again, seal the pot and select manual and set timer for 5 minutes. Release pressure using quick release. Remove lid. Stir well and serve.

NUTRITION: Calories 459 Fat 20.5 g Carbohydrates 14.9 g Protein 9.2 g

57. Greek Chicken Rice

Preparation Time: 10 minutes

Cooking Time: 14 minutes

Servings: 4

INGREDIENTS:

- 3 chicken breasts, skinless, boneless, and cut into chunks
- 1/4 fresh parsley, chopped
- 1 zucchini, sliced
- 2 bell peppers, chopped
- 1 cup rice, rinsed and drained
- 1 1/2 cup chicken broth
- 1 tbsp oregano

- 3 tbsp fresh lemon juice

- 1 tbsp garlic, minced

- 1 onion, diced

- 2 tbsp olive oil

- Pepper

- Salt

DIRECTIONS:

1. Add oil into the inner pot of instant pot and set the pot on sauté mode. Add onion and chicken and cook for 5 minutes. Add rice, oregano, lemon juice, garlic, broth, pepper, and salt and stir everything well.

2. Seal pot with lid and cook on high for 4 minutes. Once done, release pressure using quick release. Remove lid. Add parsley, zucchini, and bell peppers and stir well.

3. Seal pot again with lid and select manual and set timer for 5 minutes. Release pressure using quick release. Remove lid. Stir well and serve.

NUTRITION: Calories 500 Fat 16.5 g Carbohydrates 48 g Protein 38.7 g

58. Flavorful Chicken Tacos

Preparation Time: 10 minutes

Cooking Time: 10 minutes

Servings: 3

INGREDIENTS:

- 2 chicken breasts, skinless and boneless
- 1 tbsp chili powder
- 1/2 tsp ground cumin
- 1/2 tsp garlic powder
- 1/4 tsp onion powder
- 1/2 tsp paprika
- 4 oz can green chilis, diced
- 1/4 cup chicken broth
- 14 oz can tomato, diced
- Pepper
- Salt

DIRECTIONS:

1. Add all ingredients except chicken into the instant pot and stir well. Add chicken and stir. Seal pot with lid and cook on high for 10 minutes.
2. Once done, allow to release pressure naturally for 5 minutes then release remaining using quick release. Remove lid.
3. Remove chicken from pot and shred using a fork. Return shredded chicken to the pot and stir well. Serve and enjoy.

NUTRITION: Calories 237 Fat 8 g Carbohydrates 10.8 g Protein 30.5 g

59. Quinoa Chicken Bowls

Preparation Time: 10 minutes
Cooking Time: 6 minutes

Servings: 4

INGREDIENTS:

- 1 lb. chicken breasts, skinless, boneless, and cut into chunks
- 14 oz can chickpeas, drained and rinsed
- 1 cup olives, pitted and sliced
- 1 cup cherry tomatoes, halved
- 1 cucumber, sliced
- 2 tsp Greek seasoning
- 1 1/2 cups chicken broth
- 1 cup quinoa, rinsed and drained
- Pepper
- Salt

DIRECTIONS:

1. Add broth and quinoa into the instant pot and stir well. Season chicken with Greek seasoning, pepper, and salt and place into the instant pot.
2. Seal pot with lid and cook on high for 6 minutes. Once done, release pressure using quick release. Remove lid. Stir quinoa and chicken mixture well.
3. Add remaining ingredients and stir everything well. Serve immediately and enjoy it.

NUTRITION: Calories 566 Fat 16.4 g Carbohydrates 57.4 g Protein 46.8 g

60. Quick Chicken with Mushrooms

Preparation Time: 10 minutes

Cooking Time: 22 minutes

Servings: 6

INGREDIENTS:

- 2 lb. chicken breasts, skinless and boneless
- 1/2 cup heavy cream
- 1/3 cup water
- 3/4 lb. mushrooms, sliced
- 3 tbsp olive oil
- 1 tsp Italian seasoning
- Pepper
- Salt

DIRECTIONS:

1. Add oil into the inner pot of instant pot and set the pot on sauté mode. Season chicken with Italian seasoning, pepper, and salt.

2. Add chicken to the pot and sauté for 5 minutes. Remove chicken from pot and set aside. Add mushrooms and sauté for 5 minutes or until mushrooms are lightly brown.

3. Return chicken to the pot. Add water and stir well. Seal pot with a lid and select manual and set timer for 12 minutes.

4. Once done, release pressure using quick release. Remove lid. Remove chicken from pot and place on a plate.

5. Set pot on sauté mode. Add heavy cream and stir well and cook for 5 minutes. Pour mushroom sauce over chicken and serve.

NUTRITION: Calories 396 Fat 22.3 g Carbohydrates 2.2 g Protein 45.7 g

61. Herb Garlic Chicken

Preparation Time: 10 minutes

Cooking Time: 12 minutes

Servings: 8

INGREDIENTS:

- 4 lb. chicken breasts, skinless and boneless
- 1 tbsp garlic powder
- 2 tbsp dried Italian herb mix
- 2 tbsp olive oil
- 1/4 cup chicken stock
- Pepper
- Salt

DIRECTIONS:

1. Coat chicken with oil and season with dried herb, garlic powder, pepper, and salt. Place chicken into the instant pot. Pour stock over the chicken. Seal pot with a lid and select manual and set timer for 12 minutes.

2. Once done, allow to release pressure naturally for 5 minutes then release remaining using quick release. Remove lid. Shred chicken using a fork and serve.

NUTRITION: Calories 502 Fat 20.8 g Carbohydrates 7.8 g Protein 66.8 g

RICE, BEAN, AND GRAIN

RECIPES

62. Confetti Couscous

Preparation time: 5 minutes

Cooking time: 20 minutes

Servings: 4-6

INGREDIENTS:

- 3 tablespoons olive oil
- 1 large chopped onion
- 1 cup fresh peas
- 2 carrots, chopped
- ½ cup golden raisins
- 1 teaspoon salt
- 2 cups vegetable broth
- 2 cups couscous

DIRECTIONS:

1. Add the olive oil, onions, peas, raisins, and carrots to a skillet over medium heat. Allow to cook for 5 minutes, stirring occasionally, or until the vegetables start to soften.

2. Season with salt and pour in the vegetable broth while whisking. Bring it to a boil for about 5 minutes. Fold in the couscous and stir to combine.

3. Reduce the heat to low and cook covered for about 10 minutes, or until the couscous has absorbed the liquid completely. Using a fork to fluff the couscous and serve while warm.

NUTRITION: Calories: 515 Fat: 12.3g Carbs: 92.3g Protein: 14.2g

63. Lemon-Herbs Orzo

Preparation time: 15 minutes

Cooking time: 10 minutes

Servings: 4

INGREDIENTS:

- Orzo:
- 2 cups orzo
- ½ cup fresh basil, finely chopped
- 2 tablespoons lemon zest
- ½ cup fresh parsley, finely chopped
- Dressing:
- ½ cup extra-virgin olive oil
- 1/3 cup lemon juice
- 1 teaspoon salt
- ½ teaspoon freshly ground black pepper

DIRECTIONS:

1. Put the orzo in a large saucepan of boiling water and allow to cook for 6 minutes. Drain the orzo in a sieve and rinse well under cold running water. Set aside to cool completely.

2. When cooled, place the orzo in a large bowl. Mix in the basil, lemon zest, and parsley. Set aside.

3. Make the dressing: In a separate bowl, combine the olive oil, lemon juice, salt, and pepper. Stir to incorporate.

4. Pour the dressing into the bowl of orzo mixture and toss gently until everything is well combined. Serve immediately, or refrigerate for later.

NUTRITION: Calories: 570 Fat: 29.3g Carbs: 65.1g Protein: 11.2g

64. Mediterranean Orzo and Vegetables Pilaf

Preparation time: 15 minutes

Cooking time: 10 minutes

Servings: 6

INGREDIENTS:

- 2 cups orzo
- 1 cup Kalamata olives
- 1 pint (2 cups) cherry tomatoes, cut in half
- ½ cup fresh basil, finely chopped
- Dressing:
- ½ cup extra-virgin olive oil
- 1/3 cup balsamic vinegar

- 1 teaspoon salt

- ½ teaspoon freshly ground black pepper

DIRECTIONS:

1. Put the orzo in a large pot of boiling water and allow to cook for 6 minutes. Drain the orzo in a sieve and rinse well under cold running water. Set aside to cool completely.

2. When cooled, place the orzo in a large bowl. Add the olives, tomatoes, and basil. Toss well.

3. Mix together the olive oil, vinegar, pepper, and salt in a separate bowl. Pour the dressing into the bowl of orzo and vegetables.

4. Toss gently to mix them thoroughly. Serve chilled or at room temperature.

NUTRITION: Calories: 480 Fat: 28.3g Carbs: 48.2g Protein: 8.1g

65. Lentils and Bulgur Wheat and Browned Onions

Preparation time: 15 minutes

Cooking time: 35 minutes

Servings: 6

INGREDIENTS:

- ½ cup olive oil

- 4 large chopped onions

- 2 teaspoons salt, divided

- 2 cups brown lentils, picked over and rinsed

- 6 cups water

- 1 cup bulgur wheat
- 1 teaspoon freshly ground black pepper

DIRECTIONS:

1. Heat the olive oil in a saucepan over medium heat. Add the onions and sauté for 3 to 4 minutes until the edges are lightly browned.
2. Season with 1 teaspoon of salt. Reserve half of the cooked onions on a platter for later use.
3. Add the remaining salt, lentils, and water to the remaining onions in the saucepan. Stir to combine and cook covered for about 20 to 25 minutes, stirring occasionally.
4. Fold in the bulgur wheat and sprinkle with the black pepper. Give it a good stir and cook for 5 minutes more. Using a fork to fluff the mixture, cover, and allow to sit for 5 minutes.
5. Remove from the saucepan to six serving plates. Serve topped with the reserved cooked onions.

NUTRITION: Calories: 485 Fat: 20.4g Carbs: 59.5g Protein: 20.1g

66. Quick Spanish Rice

Preparation time: 10 minutes

Cooking time: 15 minutes

Servings: 4

INGREDIENTS:

- 2 tablespoons olive oil
- 1 medium onion, finely chopped
- 1 large tomato, finely diced

- 1 teaspoon smoked paprika
- 2 tablespoons tomato paste
- 1½ cups basmati rice
- 1 teaspoon salt
- 3 cups water

DIRECTIONS:

1. Heat the olive oil in a saucepan over medium heat. Add the onions and tomato and sauté for about 3 minutes until softened.
2. Add the paprika, tomato paste, basmati rice, and salt. Stir the mixture for 1 minute and slowly pour in the water.
3. Reduce the heat to low and allow to simmer covered for 12 minutes, stirring constantly. Remove from the heat and let it rest in the saucepan for 3 minutes. Divide the rice evenly among four serving bowls and serve.

NUTRITION: Calories: 331 Fat: 7.3g Carbs: 59.8g Protein: 6.1g

67. Rustic Lentil and Basmati Rice Pilaf

Preparation time: 15 minutes

Cooking time: 50 minutes

Servings: 6

INGREDIENTS:

- ¼ cup olive oil
- 1 large onion, chopped
- 1 teaspoon ground cumin
- 1 teaspoon salt

- 6 cups water
- 2 cups brown lentils, picked over and rinsed
- 1 cup basmati rice

DIRECTIONS:

1. Heat the olive oil in a saucepan over medium heat. Add the onions and cook for about 4 minutes until the onions are a medium golden color.
2. Turn the heat to high and add the cumin, salt, and water. Allow the mixture to boil for about 3 minutes until heated through.
3. Reduce the heat to medium-low and add the brown lentils. Allow to simmer covered for about 20 minutes until tender, stirring occasionally.
4. Add the basmati rice and stir well. Cook for 20 minutes until the rice has absorbed the liquid completely.
5. Using a fork to fluff the rice, cover, and let stand for 5 minutes. Transfer to plates and serve hot.

NUTRITION: Calories: 400 Fat: 11.3g Carbs: 59.7g Protein: 18.4g

68. Creamy Polenta with Parmesan Cheese

Preparation time: 15 minutes

Cooking time: 25 minutes

Servings: 4

INGREDIENTS:

- 3 tablespoons olive oil

- 1 tablespoon garlic, finely chopped
- 1 teaspoon salt
- 4 cups water
- 1 cup polenta
- ¾ cup Parmesan cheese, divided

DIRECTIONS:

1. In a large saucepan, heat the olive oil over medium heat. Cook the garlic for 2 minutes until fragrant. Season with 1 teaspoon salt.

2. Pour in the water and bring it to a rapid boil. Fold in the polenta and stir for 3 minutes until it begins to thicken.

3. Reduce the heat to low, cover, and allow to simmer covered for about 20 minutes, whisking constantly.

4. Add the ½ cup of the Parmesan cheese and stir to combine. Divide the polenta into four serving bowls and serve sprinkled with remaining cheese.

NUTRITION: Calories: 300 Fat: 15.8g Carbs: 27.5g Protein: 8.7g

69. Bean and Toasted Pita Salad

Preparation time: 15 minutes

Cooking time: 6 minutes

Servings: 4

INGREDIENTS:

- 3 tbsp chopped fresh mint
- 3 tbsp chopped fresh parsley

- 1 cup crumbled feta cheese
- 1 cup sliced romaine lettuce
- ½ cucumber, peeled and sliced
- 1 cup diced plum tomatoes
- 2 cups cooked pinto beans, well drained and slightly warmed
- Pepper to taste
- 3 tbsp extra virgin olive oil
- 2 tbsp ground toasted cumin seeds
- 2 tbsp fresh lemon juice
- 1/8 tsp salt
- 2 cloves garlic, peeled
- 2 6-inch whole wheat pita bread, cut or torn into bite-sized pieces

DIRECTIONS:

1. In large baking sheet, spread torn pita bread and bake in a preheated 400F oven for 6 minutes. With the back of a knife, mash garlic and salt until paste like. Add into a medium bowl.

2. Whisk in ground cumin and lemon juice. In a steady and slow stream, pour oil as you whisk continuously. Season with pepper.

3. In a large salad bowl, mix cucumber, tomatoes and beans. Pour in dressing, toss to coat well. Add mint, parsley, feta, lettuce and toasted pita, toss to mix once again and serve.

NUTRITION: Calories: 427 Protein: 17.7g Carbs: 47.3g Fat: 20.4g

70. Beans and Spinach Mediterranean Salad

Preparation time: 15 minutes

Cooking time: 15 minutes

Servings: 4

INGREDIENTS:

- 1 can (14 ounces) water-packed artichoke hearts, rinsed, drained and quartered
- 1 can (14-1/2 ounces) no-salt-added diced tomatoes, undrained
- 1 can (15 ounces) cannellini beans, rinsed and drained
- 1 small onion, chopped
- 1 tablespoon olive oil
- 1/4 teaspoon pepper
- 1/4 teaspoon salt
- 1/8 teaspoon crushed red pepper flakes
- 2 garlic cloves, minced
- 2 tablespoons Worcestershire sauce
- 6 ounces fresh baby spinach (about 8 cups)
- Additional olive oil, optional

DIRECTIONS:

1. Place a saucepan on medium high fire and heat for a minute. Add oil and heat for 2 minutes. Stir in onion and sauté for 4 minutes. Add garlic and sauté for another minute.

2. Stir in seasonings, Worcestershire sauce, and tomatoes. Cook for 5 minutes while stirring continuously until sauce is reduced.

3. Stir in spinach, artichoke hearts, and beans. Sauté for 3 minutes until spinach is wilted and other ingredients are heated through. Serve and enjoy.

NUTRITION: Calories: 187 Protein: 8.0g Carbs: 30.0g Fat: 4.0g

71. Chickpea Fried Eggplant Salad

Preparation time: 15 minutes

Cooking time: 12 minutes

Servings: 4

INGREDIENTS:

- 1 cup chopped dill
- 1 cup chopped parsley
- 1 cup cooked or canned chickpeas, drained
- 1 large eggplant, thinly sliced (no more than 1/4 inch in thickness)
- 1 small red onion, sliced in 1/2 moons
- 1/2 English cucumber, diced
- 3 Roma tomatoes, diced
- 3 tbsp Za'atar spice, divided
- oil for frying, preferably extra virgin olive oil
- Salt
- Garlic Vinaigrette Ingredients:
- 1 large lime, juice of

- 1/3 cup extra virgin olive oil

- 1–2 garlic cloves, minced

- Salt & Pepper to taste

DIRECTIONS:

1. On a baking sheet, spread out sliced eggplant and season with salt generously. Let it sit for 30 minutes. Then pat dry with paper towel.

2. Place a small pot on medium high fire and fill halfway with oil. Heat oil for 5 minutes. Fry eggplant in batches until golden brown, around 3 minutes per side.

3. Place cooked eggplants on a paper towel lined plate. Once eggplants have cooled, assemble the eggplant on a serving dish. Sprinkle with 1 tbsp of Za'atar.

4. Mix dill, parsley, red onions, chickpeas, cucumbers, and tomatoes in a large salad bowl. Sprinkle remaining Za'atar and gently toss to mix.

5. Whisk well the vinaigrette ingredients in a small bowl. Drizzle 2 tbsp of the dressing over the fried eggplant. Add remaining dressing over the chickpea salad and mix.

6. Add the chickpea salad to the serving dish with the fried eggplant. Serve and enjoy.

NUTRITION: Calories: 642 Protein: 16.6g Carbs: 25.9g Fat: 44.0g

PASTA RECIPES

72. Greek Olive and Feta Cheese Pasta

Preparation Time: 90 minutes

Cooking Time: 15 minutes

Servings:

INGREDIENTS:

- 2 cloves of finely minced fresh garlic
- 2 large tomatoes, seeded and diced
- 3 oz feta cheese, crumbled
- ½ diced red bell pepper
- 10 small-sized Greek olives, coarsely chopped and pitted
- ½ diced yellow bell pepper
- ¼ cup basil leaves, coarsely chopped
- 1 Tbsp Olive oil
- ¼ tsp hot pepper, finely chopped
- 4 ½ oz of ziti pasta

DIRECTIONS·

1. Cook pasta to a desirable point, drain it, sprinkle with olive oil, and set aside.

2. In a large bowl, mix olives, feta cheese, basil, garlic, and hot pepper. Leave for 30 minutes.

3. To the same bowl, add the cooked pasta, the bell peppers, and toss. Refrigerate for up to an hour. Toss again, then serve chilled.

NUTRITION: Calories: 235 Carbs: 27g Fat: 10g Protein: 7g

73. Beef with Tomato Spaghetti

Preparation Time: 10 minutes

Cooking Time: 20 minutes

Servings: 4

INGREDIENTS:

- 12 ounces spaghetti
- Zest and juice from 1 lemon
- 2 garlic cloves, minced
- 2 tablespoons olive oil
- 1 pound beef, ground
- Salt and black pepper to taste
- 1-pint cherry tomatoes, chopped
- 1 small red onion, chopped
- ½ cup white wine
- 2 tablespoons tomato paste
- Some basil leaves, chopped for serving
- Some parmesan, grated for serving

DIRECTIONS:

1. Put water in a large saucepan, add a pinch of salt, bring to a boil over medium-high heat, add spaghetti, cook according to instructions, drain and return pasta to pan.

2. Add lemon zest and juice and 1 tablespoon oil to pasta, toss to coat, heat up over medium heat for a couple of seconds, divide between plates and keep warm.

3. Meanwhile, heat a pan with remaining oil over medium heat, add garlic, stir and cook for 1 minute. Add beef, salt, and pepper and brown it for 4 minutes.

4. Add tomato paste and wine, stir and cook for 3 minutes. Divide beef on plates, add tomatoes, red onion, basil, and parmesan and serve.

NUTRITION: Calories: 284 Protein: 15 g Fat: 2 g Carbs: 5 g

74. Vegetarian Lasagna

Preparation Time: 15 minutes

Cooking Time: 1 hour and 15 minutes

Servings: 6

INGREDIENTS:

- 1 sweet onion, sliced thick
- 1 eggplant, sliced thick
- 2 zucchinis, sliced lengthwise
- 2 tablespoons olive oil
- 28 ounces canned tomatoes, diced & sodium free
- 1 cup quartered, canned & water packed artichokes, drained

- 2 teaspoons basil, fresh & chopped
- 2 teaspoons garlic, minced
- 2 teaspoons oregano, fresh & chopped
- 12 lasagna noodles, whole grain & no-boil
- ¼ teaspoon red pepper flakes
- ¾ cup asiago cheese, grated

DIRECTIONS:

1. Start by heating your oven to 400, and then get out a baking sheet. Line it with foil before placing it to the side.

2. Get out a large bowl and toss your zucchini, yellow squash, eggplant, onion, and olive oil, making sure it's coated well.

3. Arrange your vegetables on the baking sheet, roasting for twenty minutes. They should be lightly caramelized and tender. Chop your roasted vegetables before placing them in a bowl.

4. Stir in your garlic, basil, oregano, artichoke hearts, tomatoes, and red pepper flakes, spooning a quarter of this mixture in the bottom of a nine by thirteen baking dish.

5. Arrange four lasagna noodles over this sauce, and continue by alternating it. Sprinkle with asiago cheese on top, baking for a half hour. Allow it to cool for fifteen minutes before slicing to serve.

NUTRITION: Calories: 386 Protein: 15 g Fat: 11 g Carbs: 59 g

75. Artichokes, Olives & Tuna Pasta

Preparation Time: 15 minutes

Cooking Time: 15 minutes

Servings: 4

INGREDIENTS:

- ¼ cup chopped fresh basil
- ¼ cup chopped green olives
- ¼ tsp freshly ground pepper
- ½ cup white wine
- ½ tsp salt, divided
- 1 10-oz package frozen artichoke hearts, thawed and squeezed dry
- 2 cups grape tomatoes, halved
- 2 tbsp lemon juice
- 2 tsp chopped fresh rosemary
- 2 tsp freshly grated lemon zest
- 3 cloves garlic, minced
- 4 tbsp extra virgin olive oil, divided
- 6-oz whole wheat penne pasta
- 8-oz tuna steak, cut into 3 pieces

DIRECTIONS:

1. Cook penne pasta according to package instructions. Drain and set aside. Preheat grill to medium-high.
2. In a bowl, toss and mix ¼ tsp pepper, ¼ tsp salt, 1 tsp rosemary, lemon zest, 1 tbsp oil and tuna pieces. Grill tuna for 3 minutes per side. Allow to cool and flake into bite-sized pieces.

3. On medium fire, place a large nonstick saucepan and heat 3 tbsp oil. Sauté remaining rosemary, garlic olives, and artichoke hearts for 4 minutes

4. Add wine and tomatoes, bring to a boil and cook for 3 minutes while stirring once in a while. Add remaining salt, lemon juice, tuna pieces, and pasta.

5. Cook until heated through. To serve, garnish with basil and enjoy.

NUTRITION: Calories: 127.6 Carbs: 13g Protein: 7.2g Fat: 5.2g

76. Appetizing Mushroom Lasagna

Preparation Time: 20 minutes

Cooking Time: 75 minutes

Servings: 8

INGREDIENTS:

- ½ cup grated Parmigiano-Reggiano cheese
- No boil lasagna noodles
- Cooking spray
- ¼ cup all-purpose flour
- 3 cups reduced-fat milk, divided
- 2 tbsp chopped fresh chives, divided
- 1/3 cup less fat cream cheese
- ½ cup white wine
- 6 garlic cloves, minced and divided
- 1 ½ tbsp. Chopped fresh thyme

- ½ tsp freshly ground black pepper, divided
- 1 tsp salt, divided
- 1 package 4 oz pre-sliced exotic mushroom blend
- 1 package 8oz pre-sliced cremini mushrooms
- 1 ¼ cups chopped shallots
- 2 tbsp olive oil, divided
- 1 tbsp butter
- 1 oz dried porcini mushrooms
- 1 cup boiling water

DIRECTIONS:

1. For 30 minutes, submerge porcini in 1 cup boiling water. With a sieve, strain mushroom and reserve liquid.

2. Over the medium-high fire, melt butter on a frying pan. Mix in 2 tbsp oil and for three minutes fry shallots. Add ¼ tsp pepper, ½ tsp salt, exotic mushrooms, and cremini, cook for six minutes.

3. Stir in 3 garlic cloves and thyme, cook for a minute. Bring to a boil as you pour wine by increasing fire to high and cook until liquid evaporates around a minute.

4. Turn off fire and stir in porcini mushrooms, 1 tbsp chives, and cream cheese. Mix well.

5. On medium-high fire, place a separate medium-sized pan with 1 tbsp oil. Sauté for half a minute 3 garlic cloves.

6. Then bring to a boil as you pour 2 ¾ cups milk and reserved porcini liquid. Season with remaining pepper and salt.

7. In a separate bowl, whisk together flour and ¼ cup milk and pour into pan. Stir constantly and cook until the mixture thickens.

8. In a greased rectangular glass dish, pour and spread ½ cup of sauce, top with lasagna, top with half of the mushroom mixture and another layer of lasagna.

9. Repeat the layering process and instead of the lasagna layer, end with the mushroom mixture and cover with cheese.

10. For 45 minutes, bake the lasagna in a preheated 350F oven. Garnish with chives before serving.

NUTRITION: Calories: 268 Carbs: 29.6g Protein: 10.2g Fat: 12.6g

77. Cajun Garlic Shrimp Noodle Bowl

Preparation Time: 15 minutes

Cooking Time: 15 minutes

Servings: 2

INGREDIENTS:

- ½ teaspoon salt
- 1 onion, sliced
- 1 red pepper, sliced
- 1 tablespoon butter
- 1 teaspoon garlic granules
- 1 teaspoon onion powder
- 1 teaspoon paprika
- 2 large zucchinis, cut into noodle strips

- 20 jumbo shrimps, shells removed and deveined
- 3 cloves garlic, minced
- 3 tablespoon ghee
- A dash of cayenne pepper
- A dash of red pepper flakes

DIRECTIONS:

1. Prepare the Cajun seasoning by mixing the onion powder, garlic granules, pepper flakes, cayenne pepper, paprika, and salt. Toss in the shrimp to coat in the seasoning.
2. In a skillet, heat the ghee and sauté the garlic. Add in the red pepper and onions and continue sautéing for 4 minutes. Add the Cajun shrimp and cook until opaque. Set aside.
3. In another pan, heat the butter and sauté the zucchini noodles for three minutes. Assemble by placing the Cajun shrimps on top of the zucchini noodles.

NUTRITION: Calories: 712 Fat: 30.0g Protein: 97.8g Carbs: 20.2g

78. Mediterranean Pasta with Tomato Sauce and Vegetables

Preparation Time: 15 minutes

Cooking Time: 25 minutes

Servings: 8

INGREDIENTS:

- 8 ounces linguine or spaghetti, cooked
- 1 teaspoon garlic powder

- 1 (28 ounces) can whole peeled tomatoes, drained and sliced
- 1 tablespoon olive oil
- 1 (8 ounces) can tomato sauce
- ½ teaspoon Italian seasoning
- 8 ounces mushrooms, sliced
- 8 ounces yellow squash, sliced
- 8 ounces zucchini, sliced
- ½ teaspoon sugar
- ½ cup grated Parmesan cheese

DIRECTIONS:

1. In a medium saucepan, mix tomato sauce, tomatoes, sugar, Italian seasoning, and garlic powder. Bring to boil on medium heat. Reduce heat to low. Cover and simmer for 20 minutes.

2. In a large skillet, heat olive oil on medium-high heat. Add squash, mushrooms, and zucchini. Cook, stirring, for 4 minutes or until tender-crisp.

3. Stir vegetables into the tomato sauce. Place pasta in a serving bowl. Spoon vegetable mixture over pasta and toss to coat. Top with grated Parmesan cheese.

NUTRITION: Calories: 154 Protein: 6 g Fat: 2 g Carbs: 28 g

79. Shrimp Pasta with Rosemary Sause

Preparation Time: 10 minutes

Cooking Time: 20 minutes

Servings: 4

INGREDIENTS:

- 4 tablespoons butter
- 1 tablespoon fresh thyme
- 1 tablespoon fresh rosemary
- 10 ounces shrimp, peeled, deveined
- 3 tablespoons flour
- 25 ounces of milk, warm
- ½ onion, chopped
- 1 cup fresh parsley
- ½ cup green onion, or chives
- Salt and pepper, to taste
- 1 teaspoon nutmeg
- Juice of ½ lime
- 10 ounces pasta, cooked

DIRECTIONS:

1. Add butter, rosemary, and thyme to a large pan. Stir. Add the shrimp and cook for 3 minutes. Remove from pan and set aside.

2. Sprinkle the flour into the rosemary sauce and mix until it becomes slightly brown. Continue stirring and add the warm milk slowly. Add salt, ground nutmeg, and pepper.

3. Stir and add the chopped onion. Cook for 5 minutes. Add the green onion and fresh parsley. Remove the pan from the stove. Blend everything with a hand blender in the pan.

4. Cook until the sauce is bubbling, then turn off the heat. Add the shrimp and stir to coat in sauce. Add the lime juice. Stir in the pasta. Sprinkle with chopped parsley and serve.

NUTRITION: Calories: 225 Protein: 8 g Fat: 5 g Carbs: 14 g

80. Pesto Zucchini Noodles

Preparation Time: 10 minutes

Cooking Time: 10 minutes

Servings: 3

INGREDIENTS:

- ½ red onion, thinly sliced
- 6 cremini or white button mushrooms, thinly sliced
- 10 cherry tomatoes, halved
- 2 cloves garlic, finely minced
- 2 teaspoon olive oil
- ¼ teaspoon salt
- freshly ground black pepper, to taste
- red crushed pepper, to taste
- 1 tablespoon cashew cream, optional

DIRECTIONS:

1. On medium-high heat, heat the olive oil in a non-stick pan. Add the minced garlic, sliced mushrooms, and sliced onions. Add ¼ teaspoon salt.

2. Sauté until the veggies are cooked and tender, yet remain crispy. Set aside. Wipe down the pan with a wet napkin, then heat ¼ cup pesto.

3. Add the spiralized zucchini spaghetti and sauté on medium-high heat for 1-2 minutes. Add the sautéed mushrooms/onions and cherry tomato halves.

4. Add the remainder of the pesto and a drizzle of cashew cream if using. Sauté for 1-2 minutes, tossing frequently. Season with freshly ground black pepper and red crushed pepper.

NUTRITION: Calories: 226 Protein: 5 g Fat: 20 g Carbs: 11 g

81. Pasta with Peas

Preparation Time: 10 minutes

Cooking Time: 10 minutes

Servings: 4

INGREDIENTS:

- 2 eggs
- 1 cup frozen peas
- ½ cup Parmigiano-Reggiano cheese, grated
- 12 ounces linguini
- 1 Tbsp olive oil
- 1 onion, sliced
- Salt & pepper, to taste

DIRECTIONS:

1. In a bowl, combine the zucchini noodles with salt, pepper and the olive oil and toss well. Prepare linguini according to the package. Whisk eggs and mix in cheese.

2. Sauté onion in olive oil, then stir in peas. Add pasta to pan. Add egg mixture to the pasta and cook for another 2 min. Season with salt and pepper. Serve hot.

NUTRITION: Calories: 480 Protein: 20 g Fat: 11 g Carbs: 73 g

PIZZA RECIPES

82. Mushroom Pizza

Preparation time: 15 minutes

Cooking time: 25 minutes

Servings: 8

INGREDIENTS:

- 6 oz pizza dough
- 1 cup cremini mushrooms, chopped
- 1 cup Cheddar cheese, shredded
- 3 oz goat cheese, crumbled
- 1 tablespoon olive oil
- 1 teaspoon dried thyme
- ½ teaspoon dried oregano

DIRECTIONS:

1. Roll up the pizza dough and put it in the lined with a baking paper baking tray. Then preheat olive oil in the skillet. Add cremini mushrooms and cook them for 5 minutes.

2. Then put the mushrooms over the pizza dough. Sprinkle the mushrooms with Cheddar cheese and goat cheese. Then sprinkle the pizza with thyme and oregano. Bake the pizza at 400F for 20 minutes.

NUTRITION: Calories 223 Protein 8.2g Carbohydrates 9.9g Fat 16.8g

83. Grape Pizza

Preparation time: 15 minutes

Cooking time: 10 minutes

Servings: 4

INGREDIENTS:

- 5 oz flatbread pizza crust
- 4 oz brie cheese, crumbled
- 1/3 cup red grapes, halved, seedless
- ¼ cup fresh arugula, chopped

DIRECTIONS:

1. Put the flatbread pizza crust in the baking tray. Then put the halved red grapes on the pizza crust. Sprinkle the grapes with crumbled brie cheese and bake at 400F for 10 minutes.

NUTRITION: Calories 167 Protein 9.1g Carbohydrates 9.5g Fat 10.4g

84. Gorgonzola Pizza

Preparation time: 15 minutes

Cooking time: 12 minutes

Servings: 6

INGREDIENTS:

- 1 pizza crust
- 2 pears, sliced
- 5 oz Gorgonzola, crumbled
- 2 tablespoons cream cheese

- ½ teaspoon Italian seasonings

DIRECTIONS:

1. Spread the pizza crust with cream cheese. Then put the sliced peas on the pizza crust on one layer and sprinkle with gorgonzola and Italian seasonings. Bake the pizza at 400F for 12 minutes.

NUTRITION: Calories 160 Protein 6.5g Carbohydrates 17.3g fat 8.2g

85. Focaccia Pizza

Preparation time: 15 minutes

Cooking time: 15 minutes

Servings: 2

INGREDIENTS:

- 2 slices focaccia bread
- 2 tomatoes, sliced
- ½ teaspoon dried oregano
- 2 oz Mozzarella, sliced
- 1 teaspoon minced garlic
- 1 tablespoon tomato paste

DIRECTIONS:

1. Spread the bread with tomato paste and minced garlic. Then top the bread slices with mozzarella and tomatoes and sprinkle with dried oregano. Bake the pizzas for 5 minutes at 400F.

NUTRITION: Calories 189 Protein 12.1g Carbohydrates 22.5g Fat 6.2g

86. Pesto Pizza

Preparation time: 15 minutes

Cooking time: 20 minutes

Servings: 6

INGREDIENTS:

- 6 oz pizza dough
- 4 tablespoons pesto sauce
- 1 big tomato, sliced
- ¼ cup fresh baby spinach
- 1 tablespoon balsamic vinegar

DIRECTIONS:

1. Line the baking tray with baking paper and put the pizza dough inside. Then brush it with pesto sauce and top with tomato.
2. Bake it for 20 minutes at 400F. Then sprinkle the cooked pizza with baby spinach and balsamic vinegar.

NUTRITION: Calories 184 Protein 2.9g Carbohydrates 13.9g Fat 13.1g

87. Sweet Pizza

Preparation time: 15 minutes

Cooking time: 20 minutes

Servings: 8

INGREDIENTS:

- 8 oz pizza dough
- 2 figs, chopped

- 1 teaspoon liquid honey
- 1 cup mozzarella cheese, shredded
- ½ cup marinara sauce

DIRECTIONS:

1. Brush the pizza dough with marinara sauce and transfer in the pizza mold. Then add figs, and mozzarella.
2. Bake the pizza at 400F for 20 minutes. When the pizza is cooked, sprinkle it with liquid honey.

NUTRITION: Calories 171 Protein 3.1g Carbohydrates 18g Fat 9.8g

88. Pizza Bianca

Preparation time: 15 minutes

Cooking time: 18 minutes

Servings: 4

INGREDIENTS:

- 4 oz pizza dough
- 3 tablespoons ricotta cheese
- ½ cup Mozzarella, shredded
- 1 tablespoon olive oil
- 2 tablespoons fresh basil, chopped
- ½ teaspoon minced garlic

DIRECTIONS:

1. Roll up the pizza dough in the shape of the pizza crust. Then mix minced garlic with olive oil. Brush the pizza crust with garlic oil.

2. Then sprinkle the pizza crust with ricotta and Mozzarella cheese. Add fresh basil and transfer the pizza in the preheated to 400F oven. Cook the pizza for 18 minutes.

NUTRITION: Calories 190 Protein 4g Carbohydrates 12.9g Fat 13.7g

89. Pita Pizza

Preparation time: 15 minutes

Cooking time: 10 minutes

Servings: 8

INGREDIENTS:

- 8 whole-grain pittas
- 8 teaspoons tomato sauce
- 8 Kalamata olives, sliced
- 6 oz Provolone cheese, grated

DIRECTIONS:

1. Brush every pita with tomato sauce. Then top them with Kalamata olives and grated Provolone cheese. Bake the pita pizzas at 375F for 10 minutes.

NUTRITION: Calories 205 Protein 10.4g Carbohydrates 25g Fat 6.7g

90. Naan Bread Pizza

Preparation time: 15 minutes

Cooking time: 0 minutes

Servings: 1

INGREDIENTS:

- 1 naan bread, toasted
- 1 teaspoon hummus
- ½ cucumber, chopped
- ½ tomato, chopped
- ¼ teaspoon capers, canned

DIRECTIONS:

1. Spread the naan bread with hummus and top with cucumber, tomato, and capers. Serve.

NUTRITION: Calories 97 Protein 3.6g Carbohydrates 17.5g Fat 1.8g

91. Pepperoni Pizza Bites

Preparation time: 15 minutes

Cooking time: 10 minutes

Servings: 4

INGREDIENTS:

- 4 sandwich pepperoni slices
- 2 oz mozzarella, shredded
- 1 tablespoon marinara sauce

DIRECTIONS:

1. Arrange the pepperoni slices in the muffin molds (in the shape of the cups). Bake the pepperoni slices for 5 minutes at 400F.
2. Then add marinara sauce and shredded mozzarella in every pepperoni cup. Cook the pizza bites for 5 minutes at 400F more.

NUTRITION: Calories 173 Protein 9.1g Carbohydrates 2g Fat 13.6g

DESSERT RECIPES

92. Blueberry Frozen Yogurt

Preparation Time: 10 minutes

Cooking Time: 30 minutes

Servings: 2

INGREDIENTS:

- 1-pint blueberries, fresh
- 2/3 cup honey
- 1 small lemon, juiced and zested
- 2 cups yogurt, chilled

DIRECTIONS:

1. In a saucepan, combine the blueberries, honey, lemon juice, and zest.
2. Heat over medium heat and allow to simmer for 15 minutes while stirring constantly.
3. Once the liquid has reduced, transfer the fruits in a bowl and allow to cool in the fridge for another 15 minutes.
4. Once chilled, mix together with the chilled yogurt.

NUTRITION: Calories per serving: 233; Carbs: 52.2g; Protein: 3.5 g; Fat: 2.9g

93. Deliciously Cold Lychee Sorbet

Preparation Time: 10 minutes

Cooking Time: 5 minutes

Servings: 2

INGREDIENTS:

- 2 cups fresh lychees, pitted and sliced
- 2 tablespoons honey
- Mint leaves for garnish

DIRECTIONS:

1. Place the lychee slices and honey in a food processor
2. Pulse until smooth.
3. Pour in a container and place inside the fridge for at least two hours.
4. Scoop the sorbet and serve with mint leaves.

NUTRITION: Calories per serving: 151; Carbs: 38.9g; Protein: 0.7g; Fat: 0.4

94. Tostadas

Preparation Time: 15 minutes

Cooking Time: 15 minutes

Servings: 2

INGREDIENTS:

- ½ white onion, diced
- 1 tomato, chopped
- 1 cucumber, chopped

- 1 tablespoon fresh cilantro, chopped
- ½ jalapeno pepper, chopped
- 1 tablespoon lime juice
- 6 corn tortillas
- 1 tablespoon canola oil
- 2 oz. Cheddar cheese, shredded
- ½ cup white beans, canned, drained
- 6 eggs
- ½ teaspoon butter
- ½ teaspoon Sea salt

DIRECTIONS:

1. Make Pico de Galo: in the salad bowl combine together diced white onion, tomato, cucumber, fresh cilantro, and jalapeno pepper.
2. Then add lime juice and a ½ tablespoon of canola oil. Mix up the mixture well. Pico de Galo is cooked.
3. After this, preheat the oven to 390F.
4. Line the tray with baking paper.
5. Arrange the corn tortillas on the baking paper and brush with remaining canola oil from both sides.
6. Bake the tortillas for 10 minutes or until they start to be crunchy.
7. Chill the cooked crunchy tortillas well.
8. Meanwhile, toss the butter in the skillet.
9. Crack the eggs in the melted butter and sprinkle them with sea salt.

10. Fry the eggs until the egg whites become white (cooked). Approximately for 3-5 minutes over the medium heat.

11. After this, mash the beans until you get puree texture.

12. Spread the bean puree on the corn tortillas.

13. Add fried eggs.

14. Then top the eggs with Pico de Galo and shredded Cheddar cheese.

NUTRITION: Calories 246, Fat 11.1, Fiber 4.7, Carbs 24.5, Protein 13.7

95. Mediterranean Baked Apples

Preparation Time: 10 minutes

Cooking Time: 25 minutes

Servings: 2

INGREDIENTS:

- pounds apples, peeled and sliced
- Juice from ½ lemon
- A dash of cinnamon

DIRECTIONS:

1. Preheat the oven to 2500F
2. Line a baking sheet with parchment paper then set aside.
3. In a medium bowl, apples with lemon juice and cinnamon
4. Place the apples on the parchment paper-lined baking sheet
5. Bake for 25 minutes until crisp.

NUTRITION: Calories per serving: 90; Carbs: 23.9g; Protein: 0.5g; Fat: 0.3g

96. Pizza with Sprouts

Preparation Time: 10 minutes

Cooking Time: 10 minutes

Servings: 2

INGREDIENTS:

- ½ cup wheat flour, whole grain
- 2 tablespoons butter, softened
- ¼ teaspoon baking powder
- ¾ teaspoon salt
- 5 oz. chicken fillet, boiled
- 2 oz. Cheddar cheese, shredded
- 1 teaspoon tomato sauce
- 1 oz. bean sprouts

DIRECTIONS:

1. Make the pizza crust: mix up together wheat flour, butter, baking powder, and salt. Knead the soft and non-sticky dough. Add more wheat flour if needed.
2. Leave the dough for 10 minutes to chill.
3. Then place the dough on the baking paper. Cover it with the second baking paper sheet.
4. Roll up the dough with the help of the rolling pin to get the round pizza crust.
5. After this, remove the upper baking paper sheet.
6. Transfer the pizza crust in the tray.
7. Spread the crust with tomato sauce.

8. Then shred the chicken fillet and arrange it over the pizza crust.

9. Add shredded Cheddar cheese.

10. Bake pizza for 20 minutes at 355F.

11. Then top the cooked pizza with bean sprouts and slice into the servings.

NUTRITION: Calories 157, Fat 8.8, Fiber 0.3, Carbs 8.4, Protein 10.5

97. Banana Quinoa

Preparation Time: 10 minutes

Cooking Time: 12 minutes

Servings: 2

INGREDIENTS:

- 1 cup quinoa
- 2 cup milk
- 1 teaspoon vanilla extract
- 1 teaspoon honey
- 2 bananas, sliced
- ¼ teaspoon ground cinnamon

DIRECTIONS:

1. Pour milk in the saucepan and add quinoa.

2. Close the lid and cook it over the medium heat for 12 minutes or until quinoa will absorb all liquid.

3. Then chill the quinoa for 10-15 minutes and place in the serving mason jars.

4. Add honey, vanilla extract, and ground cinnamon.

5. Stir well.

6. Top quinoa with banana and stir it before serving.

NUTRITION: Calories 279, Fat 5.3, Fiber 4.6, Carbs 48.4, Protein 10.7

98. Hearty Berry Oats

Preparation Time: 10 minutes

Cooking Time: 10 minutes

Servings: 2

INGREDIENTS:

- 11/2 cups whole-grain rolled or quick cooking oats (not instant)
- 3/4 cup fresh blueberries, raspberries, or blackberries, or a combination
- 2 teaspoons honey
- 2 tablespoons walnut pieces

DIRECTIONS:

1. Prepare the whole-grain oats according to the package directions and divide between 2 deep bowls
2. In a small microwave-safe bowl, heat the berries and honey for 30 seconds. Top each bowl of oatmeal with the fruit mixture. Sprinkle the walnuts over the fruit and serve hot.

NUTRITION: Calories 246, Fat 11.1, Fiber 4.7, Carbs 24.5, Protein 13.7

99. Cherry Almond Baked Oatmeal Cups

Preparation Time: 10 minutes

Cooking Time: 10 minutes

Servings: 2

INGREDIENTS:

- ½ cup gluten-free old-fashioned oats
- 2 tablespoons sliced almonds
- Pinch salt
- ¾ cup milk
- ½ teaspoon almond extract
- ½ teaspoon vanilla
- 1 egg, beaten
- 2 tablespoons maple syrup
- 1 cup frozen cherries, thawed
- Ricotta cheese (optional, for topping)
- Greek yogurt (optional, for topping)

DIRECTIONS:

1. Preheat the oven to 350°F and set the rack to the middle position. Oil two 8-ounce ramekins and place them on a baking sheet.
2. In a medium bowl, combine all of the ingredients and mix well. Spoon half of the mixture into each ramekin.
3. Bake for 35 to 45 minutes, or until the oats are set and a knife inserted into the middle comes out clean. They will be soft but should not be runny.
4. Let the baked oats cool for 5 to 10 minutes. Top with ricotta cheese or plain Greek yogurt, if desired.

NUTRITION: Calories 246, Fat 11.1, Fiber 4.7, Carbs 24.5, Protein 13.7

100. Berry Smoothie

Preparation Time: 10 minutes

Cooking Time: 10 minutes

Servings: 2

INGREDIENTS:

- 1/2 cup vanilla low-fat Greek yogurt
- 1/4 cup low-fat milk'
- 1/2 cup fresh or frozen blueberries or strawberries (or a combination)
- 6 to 8 ice cubes

DIRECTIONS:

1. Place the Greek yogurt, milk, and berries in a blender and blend until the berries are liquefied. Add the ice cubes and blend on high until thick and smooth. Serve immediately.

NUTRITION: Calories per serving: 90; Carbs: 23.9g; Protein: 0.5g; Fat: 0.3g

101. Classic Fig Clafoutis

Preparation Time: 35 minutes

Cooking Time: 0 minutes

Servings: 2

INGREDIENTS

- 2 large eggs

- 1/4 cup granulated sugar

- 2 tablespoons honey

- A pinch of grated nutmeg

- A pinch of flaky salt

- 1/3 cup all-purpose flour

- 1 tablespoon unsalted butter, at room temperature

- 1/4 cup whole milk

- 1/2 cup double cream

- 1/4 cup cognac

- 1 teaspoon orange zest, finely grated

- 8 figs, halved

DIRECTIONS

1. Begin by preheating your oven to 350 degrees F.

2. In a mixing dish, thoroughly combine the eggs, sugar, honey, nutmeg, and salt.

3. Gradually stir in the flour and beat until creamy and smooth. Whisk in the butter, milk, double cream, cognac, and orange zest. Mix again to combine well.

4. Divide the batter into four lightly greased ramekins.

5. Top with the fresh figs and bake in the preheated oven for about 40 minutes until the clafoutis is golden at the edges. Bon appétit!

NUTRITION: Calories: 328; Fat: 10.4g; Carbs: 45.3g; Protein: 6.3g

CONCLUSION

We are glad that you have reached the end of this book.

If you take anything away, remember to choose a day and take the time. It may seem like you are spending a lot of time cooking but remember that you will be saving that cooking and prepping time through your whole week. Now, you can focus on what you will spend all of this extra time doing! Perhaps it will be taking that exercise class you've been thinking about or some quality family time.

Hopefully, you have found at least one recipe within these chapters you are excited to try. Whether you are vegan, vegetarian, or eat everything, there is a recipe out there for you. As I said before, try to start simple.

Mediterranean diet is not just a dietary adjustment, but a complete lifestyle change. In order to correctly emulate that, we must improve not only our diet, but our physical activity as well. The public of the Mediterranean combined exercise into their routine repeatedly, and it's significant that we try and do the equivalent. Weight loss can only occur if you are following a calorie deficit diet. Even if the Mediterranean diet is easy to follow in the sense that it doesn't require counting carbs or calories, it's still important you're aware of your portion size, snacking, and caloric intake if you want lose weight. That can only happen if you're burning off more calories than what you're taking in!

The Mediterranean diet is all about lifestyle that should be enjoyed. with both pleasure and health in mind. The Mediterranean's attitude of living life with equal measure of health and pleasure paves the way for a more balanced and happy living.

To majority of people residing in the city, when you say physical activity, it's all about going to the gym using gym equipment and machines. In the Mediterranean region, it is a different story.

Daily life is set up to naturally require more activity and calorie expenditure. Urban and commercial areas are built in historic centers that preceded the invention of cars. Driving and parking in them is difficult, which necessitates a greater deal of walking.

In order to enjoy and reap the rewards of the Mediterranean diet, followers need to add enjoyable activities into their daily lives.

Good luck!

CPSIA information can be obtained
at www.ICGtesting.com
Printed in the USA
BVHW090325230221
600781BV00006B/789